BRIDGING MODERN SKINCARE WITH AYURVEDA

Understanding Integrated Dermatology

DR. AMAN SHARMA

Integrative Dermatology

Decoding Disease Patterns and Treatment Option

DEDICATED TO

The supreme consciousness which moves and guides us. All the healers of the past, present and future.
To my loving wife, kids, parents and grandparents for not only providing the support but for helping me in being what and where I am today.

ACKNOWLEDGEMENT

Writing a medical book is a team effort that includes not just the author but also others whose contributions affect the final product. I'd like to express my deepest gratitude and appreciation to everyone who played a critical role in making this book a reality.

First and foremost, I would like to convey my heartfelt thanks to **Ms. Sachi Shukla**, the content writer, for her devotion, knowledge, and relentless efforts in developing the substance of this book. Sachi's dedication to explaining complicated medical ideas with clarity and precision has been useful. This book would not have acquired the degree of accessibility and comprehensibility that it does now without her meticulous work.

I'd also like to acknowledge the entire editorial and publishing team for their professionalism, persistent support, and contribution to turning this work into a polished and well-structured publication.

I am grateful to my colleagues and mentors for their advice and ideas, which have enhanced the content's clinical relevance and real-world applicability. Their knowledge has served as a beacon of light during this trip. I cannot thank my family and friends enough for their solid support and understanding over the many hours spent researching and writing. Your faith in me was a continual source of inspiration for me.

I owe a debt of appreciation to the innumerable patients who have inspired and taught me throughout the years. I will be eternally grateful to you for providing the framework and purpose for this work.

Last but not least, I would like to thank the readers of this work. This book was developed in response to your need for information, dedication to the medical industry, and desire to improve healthcare. I hope it helps you in your goals.

Thank you everyone who has contributed to the production of this book. Your combined efforts have made this attempt feasible, and I am grateful.

Sincerely,

Dr. Aman Sharma

DISCLAIMER

The exclusive goal of this book is to impart knowledge and information. It is not intended to replace expert medical guidance, diagnosis, or care.

This book's content is meant to serve as basic information only; it is not intended to take the place of customized, expert medical advice. When in doubt about a medical problem, never hesitate to consult your doctor or another trained healthcare professional. Never ignore medical advice from professionals or put off getting it because of something you've read in this book.

Based on research and general understanding at the time of writing, the material is presented. Since medical knowledge and procedures are always changing, what is thought to be safe and correct now might not be in the future.

Any information or suggestions included in this book are used entirely at your own risk. Any direct, indirect, special, or consequential damages arising from the use of the material included in this book are not the responsibility of the writers or publishers. Any decisions you make about your health, wellbeing, or medical care must be discussed with a licensed healthcare provider.

To sum up, this book does not serve as a replacement for expert medical advice or care. For appropriate guidance and treatment for any health-related issues or diseases, it is necessary that you consult with a medical professional

INDEX

Part 1: Understanding Integrative Medicine

Part 2: Understanding and Managing Dermatological Conditions

Note for the Book's Second Volume: We are going to explore a number of important health and wellbeing-related subjects in the next edition of this book. Among these topics are:

- Autoimmunity and Psoriasis
- Type-2 Diabetes reversal and weight balance
- Blood Pressure reversal
- Sleep hygiene
- App based body type analysis and its application to customized wellness.

BOOK INTRODUCTION

An amazing fusion of conventional knowledge and cutting-edge technology has sparked a revolutionary shift in skincare in a world where everyone strives for beautiful, healthy skin. Enter the fascinating world of "Bridging Modern Skin Care with Ayurveda: Understanding Integrated Medicine," a trip that not only spans the gap between two seemingly unrelated healthcare spheres but also reveals the path for holistic well-being

This book serves as your entryway to the synthesis of age-old Ayurvedic knowledge with cutting-edge dermatological concepts, where the distinctions between tradition and innovation are blurred to provide a harmonious approach to skincare. We welcome you to embark on a transforming journey via these pages, empowering you with significant insights and advice for anyone aiming to find all-encompassing answers to their skin difficulties.

Part 1: Clarifying Our investigation is built on the fundamental principle of integrative medicine. We set off on a discovery quest in these chapters. We start by dissecting the basic foundation of integrative medicine, exposing its fundamental ideas, investigating its safety, and examining its cost-effectiveness. You will get a deep understanding of why integrative medicine stands as a ray of hope in today's complex health care landscape as you read through these pages.

Part 2: Understanding and Managing Dermatological Conditions digs even farther into this fascinating synthesis of old wisdom and modern expertise. In this part, we move our emphasis to the complex realm of skin issues that many people face. We present a thorough explanation of what causes various dermatological disorders, how they appear, and, most importantly, how integrative techniques can guide successful care.

Here, you'll go on a voyage of discovery and empowerment, obtaining the information and skills you need to make educated decisions about your skin's health. With this newfound knowledge, you will be better able to nurture skin that expresses not just beauty but also health and energy.

The adventure starts here, where tradition meets innovation and old knowledge meets scientific progress. Welcome to "Bridging Modern Skin Care with Ayurveda: Understanding Integrated Medicine." Your journey to comprehensive skin health and well-being is waiting for you.

PART 1:
'UNDERSTANDING INTEGRATED MEDICINE'

CHAPTER 1
WHAT IS INTEGRATIVE MEDICINE?

Integrative medicine combines various treatments and lifestyle changes to treat and heal the person as a whole.

Glowing from Within: The Power of Integrative Dermatology

The developing area of Integrative Dermatology stems from allopathic medicine's new era learning. It is also an extension of ancient wisdom's essential concepts and time-tested methods of existence. To put it simply, integrative

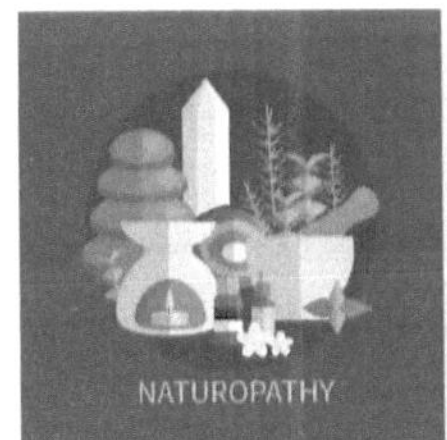

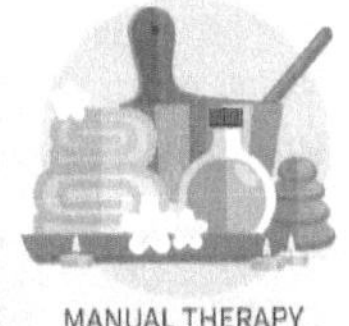

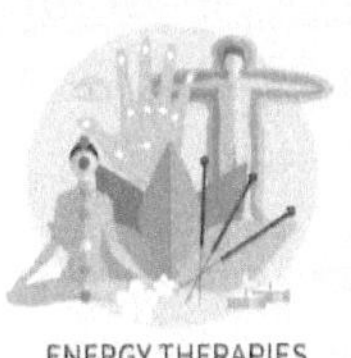

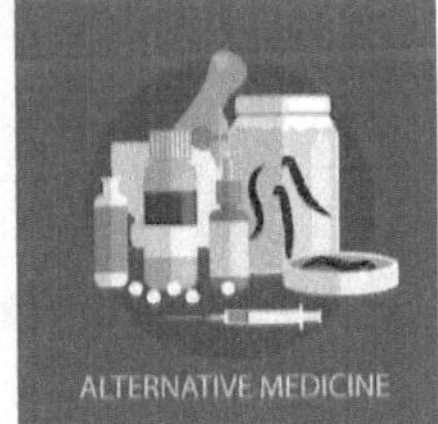

dermatology is a philosophy that combines the finest of laboratory-tested, evidence-based facts and breakthroughs in western medicine with time-tested methods of traditional wisdom. Integrative dermatology represents a paradigm change in how we see health and illness.

On the physician's end, there is a shift in patient care beginning with the patient, the doctor's chamber, history taking, counseling, and management and therapeutic choices.

The practice and knowledge of this also nudges us toward a universally accepting attitude, to agree or at least be open to the possibility that alternative medicine, particularly Ayurveda and therapeutic yoga, may contain vital solutions in illness management and enhancing treatment outcomes.

We have been indoctrinated in allopathy to reject tradition and to dismiss therapy approaches such as ethnobotanicals and yoga. All of this has occurred throughout the years under the pretext of being "scientific" and adhering to a "evidence-based approach." The notion of "evidence generation" and following evidence-based medicine has its own set of flaws, as demonstrated by several respectable and substantial research, and it has the potential to mislead the physician community.

A real scientific mind will not dismiss any system of medicine, Ayurvedic or Yogic, without first putting it to the test.

There have been several articles in the last ten years or so that support the use of different phytoceuticals, botanicals, and plant extracts in the treatment of symptoms and illness. There has been a lot of scientific research done on therapeutic yoga and breathing practices for illness prevention and treatment.

Integrative medicine attempts to integrate all of these discoveries together and give them a small, if not equal, place on the therapeutic management ladder of physicians, not only in dermatology but across disciplines.
Let us consider a tiny instance of boils and abscesses and how integrative medicine techniques might help. To improve treatment results, a standard approach will be to utilize oral and topical antibiotics (which are highly needed), as well as anti-inflammatories and enzyme-based anti-inflammatories. An allopath may advise you to make lifestyle and dietary adjustments, such as cutting back on sugar. With this strategy, we are seeing a lot of recurrences. It is not only a recurrent expenditure, but there is also the potential of germ resistance.

The Integrative Medicine method will incorporate Ayurvedic and yoga concepts, as well as habits, daily routine, nutrition, mental attitude, sleep history, stress, "unmaad," and bowel motions. Depending on the body type and dermatological problem, "Panchakarma" = Bio-cleaning specific procedures may be necessary, but in general, a bowel cleaning therapy will be advised, which may operate by correcting 'dysbiosis' in the gut, which affects immunity and metabolism.

Yogic practices have spread across countries and cultures, becoming an integral part of daily life.

The yogic method, for example, will consider how the patient breathes. Attention and practice in breathing will add no expense but will improve oxygenation and medical therapy results.

Don't allow your thinking to dismiss this overly simplified example. All of this is completely possible and requires only a shift in thinking, as well as openness and desire. All that is required is a properly scientific mind.

It is being done at some of the world's most prestigious institutes, where Ayurvedic, yoga, and traditional Chinese medical concepts and practices are being incorporated.

Even as we read, more proof is being gathered, and more individuals are benefiting from the shift in mindset. With each "pathy" abandoning its ego, an amalgamation towards oneness in healing rather than treating is being built.

PRINCIPLES OF INTEGRATED DERMATOLOGY:

Integrative dermatology is based on many fundamental principles:

Patient-centered care: Integrative dermatology places the patient at the center of care, focusing on their own requirements, preferences, and values. Patients are included in their treatment regimens, and they are encouraged to take an active role in their skin health journey.

Overall examination: Integrative dermatology is a holistic examination that looks at the patient's health, lifestyle, nutrition, stress levels, environment, and everything else. This thorough examination aids in determining the underlying cause of skin problems.

Individual Treatment Plan: Treatment plans are customized for each individual, combining standard skin treatments like topical creams, drugs, and procedures with complementary therapies including diet, stress medicine, acupuncture, herbs, and lifestyle changes.

Integrating evidence-based strategies: Integrative Dermatology includes evidence-based techniques from both conventional and alternative medicine, ensuring that therapies are supported by scientific research and shown efficacy.

They emphasize prevention: preventing integrative dermatology is critical. The emphasis is on teaching patients on good skin care techniques, diet, stress management, and other preventative methods to preserve skin health and avoid future problems.

Collaborated care: Participating dermatologists frequently work with other healthcare specialists such as dietitians, psychologists, acupuncturists, and naturopaths to build a multidisciplinary team that provides a comprehensive approach to skin health.

Adjuvant treatments are included:

Integrative dermatology includes, but is not limited to, the following complementary therapies:

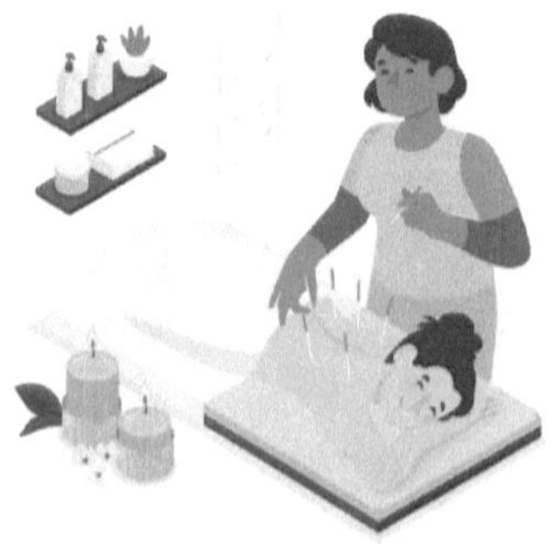

Nutrition and diet: Identification and management of dietary factors that might lead to skin disorders.

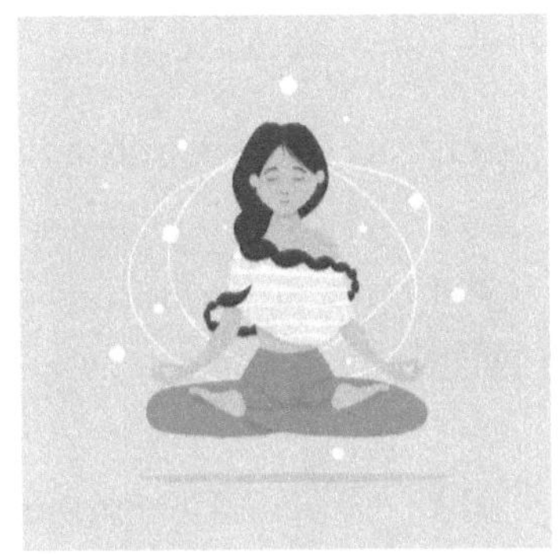

Mind-body practices: Using techniques like meditation, yoga, and biofeedback to reduce stress, which can have an impact on skin health.

Ayurveda: The use of Ayurvedic methods and medicines to balance the body and enhance skin health.

Traditional Chinese Medicine (TCM): Acupuncture, herbs, and cupping are used in Traditional Chinese Medicine (TCM) to balance the body's qi and treat skin disorders.

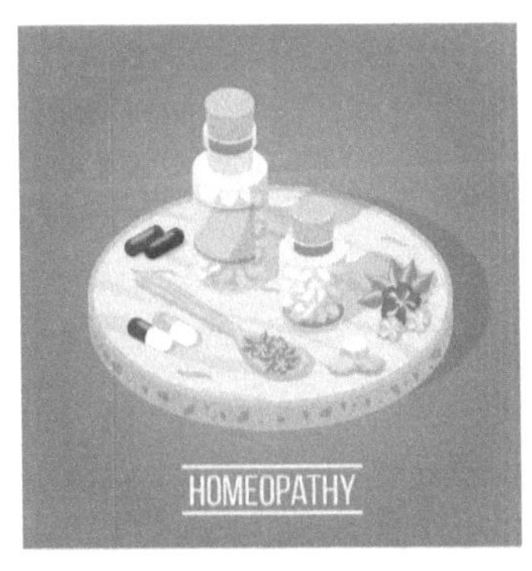

Homeopathy: The use of a mixture of homeopathic medicines to treat skin diseases depending on a patient's symptom profile.

Integrative Dermatology is a new and innovative approach to skin health that recognizes the numerous linkages between the skin and other elements of one's life. Traditional dermatology, including alternative therapy, has prioritized total health.

WHY INTEGRATIVE DERMATOLOGY?

With the development of open access technologies, publications, and an explosion of knowledge, we have seen a shift in how we see sickness. Patients and doctors are equally affected by the paradigm shift.

Despite being just roughly 100 years old, modern allopathic medicine has advanced by leaps and bounds.

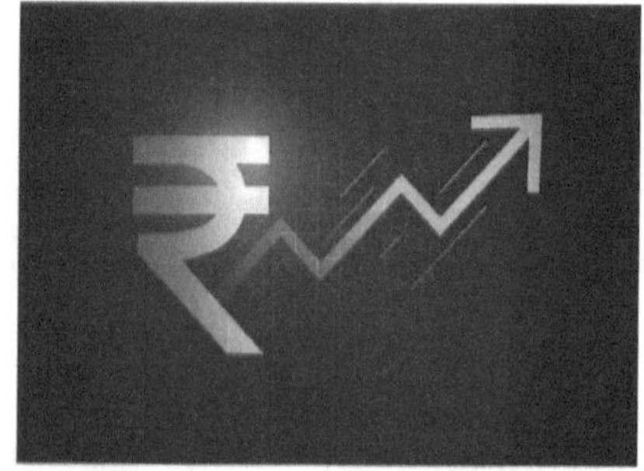

However, there are many loopholes, and the healthcare infrastructure is not only incredibly expensive (particularly in the West), but it is also collapsing across the world. The infrastructure is reliant, costly, and extremely unstable.

Furthermore, the pharmacology lobby has earned a bad reputation for being a part of the machinery that has converted people's health into a profitable business model. Awareness of all of this, as well as the reality that everyone suffering from any condition wants to lessen their "pill load" or be "fully healed" and be free of all medications.

This might be a conscious or subconscious urge.This simply demonstrates an unmet need for better patient outcomes, and it is from this need that the notion of integrative medicine arose.

Integrative medicine is a holistic remedial approach that treats numerous symptoms or cures a disease, and it is the solution to many issues. It is a collection of several linked sciences, each with its own concepts and methodologies, with the purpose of finding a solution to a specific problem.

Integrative medicine is a concept and set of management strategies aimed only at improving illness outcomes. A method in which we see the disease as a symptom-outcome rather than the problem itself. And when it comes to the origins and birth of integrative medicine, the vast and uncharted territory of integrative dermatology cannot be far behind.

The skin, being the biggest organ of the body, is an exact representation of a person's system. According to current knowledge and greater understanding, skin is a neuroendocrine organ that responds to a variety of circulating hormones and chemicals in the body.

Cosmetologist

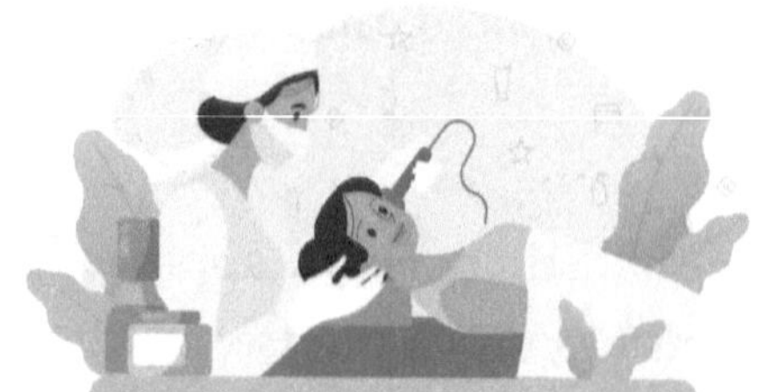

The importance of skin lies not only in its functions and as the biggest organ, but also in its aesthetic and good looks.

It has been repeatedly demonstrated that many skin issues have a significant influence on quality of life, anxiety, and psychology. The feel-good element of skin attractiveness is a crucial, but often overlooked, truth.

As a result, cosmetic dermatology has grown into a multibillion-dollar industry. The emphasis is mostly on looking nice and feeling great. The emphasis has switched from addressing diseases to improving the appearance, feel, and texture of the skin.

The methods and talents in this profession have grown by leaps and bounds, and just recently, with a greater grasp of lifestyle issues and "wellness elements," the aesthetic sector is delving far deeper than simply the skin and managing individuals more holistically.

Integrative dermatological ideas and practices not only help us better understand the "root causes" of aesthetic disorders, but they may also help us considerably improve patient outcomes.

We can understand this with a simple example of Dandruff. Dandruff is a common dermatological condition marked by the shedding of dead skin cells from the scalp. While it is frequently ascribed to a yeast accumulation on the scalp and the skin's immunological reactivity in areas rich in oil glands, it is critical to realize that a variety of variables can worsen this illness. Excess sugar consumption can promote yeast development, while mineral deficiency might harm the health of the scalp. Acidic meals can also disturb the pH balance of the scalp, exacerbating the problem.

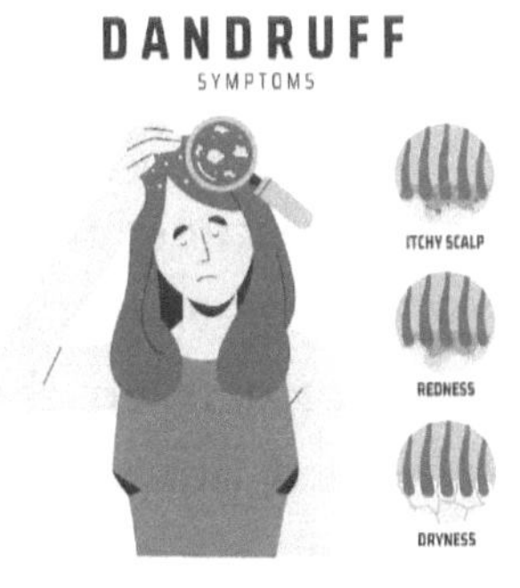

Integrative wellness methods promote the notion of lifespan while providing a comprehensive solution to improve the outcomes of aesthetic and cosmetic dermatology. Integrative health can give long-term relief by treating not just the surface symptoms but also the underlying causes of dandruff. This includes a well-balanced diet low in sugar and high in key minerals, as well as stress management strategies and tailored skincare regimens. Such a thorough method not only eliminates dandruff but also promotes general skin health, making it an essential component in achieving long-term attractiveness and well-being. Adopting these measures can result in not only a glowing complexion but also a healthier, more meaningful life, stressing the relevance of longevity in the field of cosmetic dermatology.

SO WHAT DOES INTEGRATIVE DERMATOLOGY STAND FOR? WHICH "PATHY"?

This question arises often in everyone's thoughts. The basic core of this question is that our prior experiences and impacts on the conscious mind have colored and confused our judgments. We wish to compartmentalize and split the notions with which we are already familiar. We want to place Integrative Dermatology in a box that we've already made. To establish a new place, a new for an unknown and uncharted terrain, in our imaginations, is always greeted with opposition.

One of the main reasons for writing this article is to dispel this misconception regarding integrative dermatology. Unlearn and learn, learn again, afresh, again, refresh or revitalize the dwindling trust in therapies. Realizing that it is quite possible to have a method of treatment that goes beyond simply treating, that can aid in healing from within, that can aid in fully knowing ourselves so that we may heal ourselves.

To do this, we must remove those preconceptions and break the competition of Allopathy, Ayurveda, and Yoga practitioners; ego and therapy cannot coexist. Allow competitiveness and ego to fade into a sea of global love and equality. And, with the ego removed, the potion that emerges is an equimolar blend of everything centered on the single pivot of enhancing treatment results and living a healthier, happier, and more tranquil existence.

I've always compared the practice of various medical systems, such as ayurveda, yoga, and allopathy, to different faiths. On the surface, there is a lot of dispute and disagreement. The "gods" did not battle and dispute like the founders of other religious groups. It is their adherents, the practitioners of the faiths, who are at odds. Similarly, practitioners of diverse therapeutic systems are frequently at odds with one another. The therapy systems are all focused on the same goal: enhanced patient treatment outcomes.

So integrated dermatology belongs to individuals in need of healing, not to any one system of "pathy." It exists solely to improve treatment outcomes utilizing everything known to man, as safely and scientifically as feasible.

DOES INTEGRATIVE DERMATOLOGY APPLY TO PREVENTION OR TREATMENT OF EXISTING PROBLEMS TOO?

The mere emergence of this query in our minds indicates that we have not fully comprehended our current condition of being.

Being totally healthy is more than just being free of sickness. Health is more than just a physical, mental, and emotional well-being; it is also more than just the absence of sickness. Importantly, health also includes spiritual wellness. Though a full examination of the latter is beyond the scope of this paper, it is far too crucial to overlook. But, before we move on, it's vital to note that spiritual health should not be confused with one's beliefs, religion, or ritualistic heritage.

Once we ingest this condition of health, which is constantly in flux, a continual endeavor to be healthy, to stay in balance, the subject of treating or avoiding sickness disappears. It is a voyage, and we may require more than just a mode of transportation; we may require all supporting components, tools, and locations of rest and reference for the journey.

Integrative dermatology is the path to take. Though the destination appears to be aimed at improving treatment outcomes from one dimension, the destination from another dimension may be to maintain a continuous state of balance that we may choose to call health, or in ayurveda we call it a balance of all three "doshas," in Chinese medicine we call it a balance of "yin and yang," and in Yoga it is called a balance of "ida and pingala with *sushumna* activated."

Whatever words we use to describe it, it will ultimately remain a journey to be undertaken in order to remain in balance to answer this question of prevention treatment at a more gross and course level, in an overly simplistic but factual way, integrative dermatology can treat and prevent with equal ease in most scenarios, when we choose tools at our disposal wisely and appropriately. We mean allopathy, Ayurveda, and yogic treatments when we say instruments.

As an example, if we are dealing with mental issues, chronic lifestyle disorders, and so on, the combination of ayurveda, allopathy, and yogic treatment will be different, say 1:1:1. And, if we are dealing with a habitual sleep disturbance, the mix may vary based on the individual's personality as well as the physician's openness, experience, and comfort level in employing his blend of numerous possibilities. When dealing with a sudden shock or accident, the subject of mixing between Ayurveda and allopathy usually does not arise, at least not at first. In this case, we may employ a 1:0:0 ratio in the acute and early phases, and after stabilization, the blend may shift to 0:1:2

or 0:2:1, depending on the nature of the patients' difficulties and residual sequelae.

With this insight, instead of asking where to apply integrative dermatological principles and practices, let us take the first step and progress towards (if not all of the problems), but a few problems with the integrative dermatology approach.

BEFORE PUTTING IT TO PRACTICE, IS IT SAFE?

We all want the best for our family, whether it's food, medication, transportation, or anything else. Nobody wants to jeopardize their safety. In general, your healthcare worker, doctor, therapist, or nurse practitioner will be the last to jeopardize your safety and betray their profession. So practically all healthcare practitioners are aware of the idea that they should desire well for all of their patients and typically go out of their way to follow safety precautions.

Let us first be scientific in our approach to answering this fundamental question. Let us begin by asking, what are the elements in the practice of integrative medicine, what it embraces, and what may be done that is potentially dangerous?

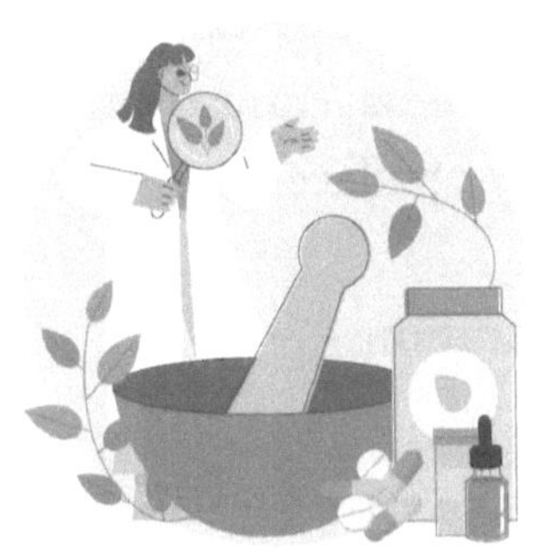

In general, when we choose to follow an integrated dermatological treatment plan, the percentage of these substances might range from zero to maximum utilization of one therapy technique.

Here is a list of the ingredients:

1. External applications such as creams, gels, lotions, cleansers, medicated creams, pastes=Ubtan, medicated oils and Ghees, and so on.

2. Allopathic pills, capsules, vitamins, antibiotics, blood pressure medicine, and diabetic medication.

3. Traditional ayurveda polyherbal formulations (made up of more than one plant)

4. Traditional Ayurvedic/herbal/botanical single herbs or mixtures, commonly used as dietary supplements in the West.

5. Bio-Cleansing/rinsing cavities, sinuses, intestines, etc. Ayurvedic or naturopathy/yogic detox procedures, such as Panchakarma in Ayurveda.

6. Allopathic procedures include lasers, surgeries, and cosmetic aesthetic interventions that can be minimally invasive, such as an injection or endoscopy, or highly invasive, such as heart surgery or a facelift.

7. Yoga-based lifestyle modifications

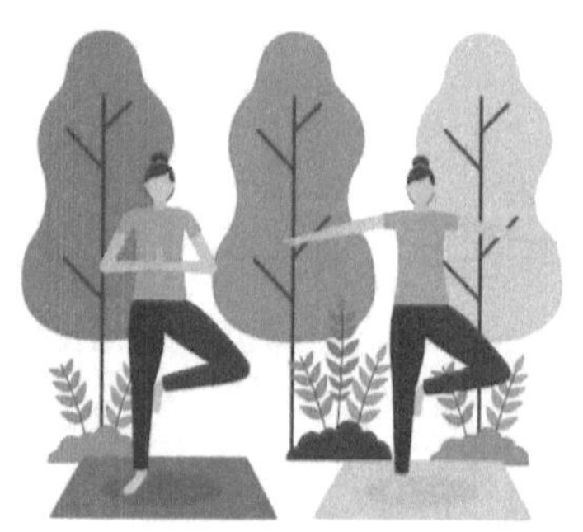

Yoga-based exercise for the body, mind, and breathing exercises (not necessarily Pranayama as we currently understand it), meditation, chanting of certain mantras, and so on. In addition to this, "Mudra" plays a significant role in health and sickness.

8. Dietetic counseling, particularly Ayurvedic measures, is especially helpful in dermatology.

Now, with an open mind, accept the safety of each concerned party, but close our eyes and halt for a second at each alternative.

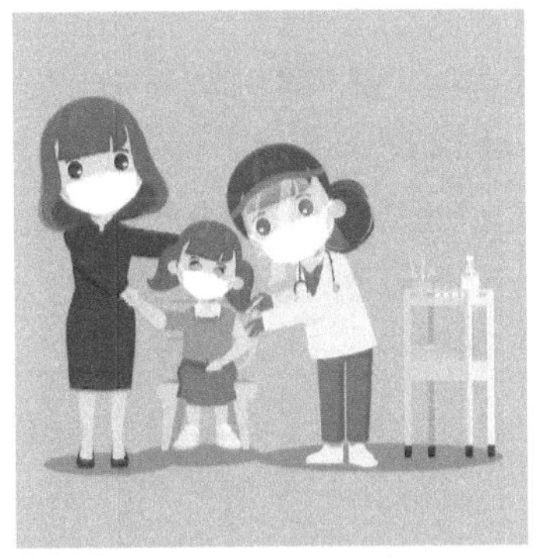

Almost all of us have been exposed to allopathic medicine in some way, whether it was through supplements or vitamin injections. Even vitamin B12 and antioxidant injections like glutathione have uncommon but potentially fatal side effects. The probable risks, etc., are all explicitly stated, and we make an informed, consented-upon decision.

Even vaccination shots for children have a major impact on their immune systems and are known to have long-term effects or even life-threatening problems. Vaccines, on the other hand, are part of national health programs, and some are even required. Despite the fact that this is common knowledge, we must remember to be grateful that vaccinations have been able to eradicate illnesses such as smallpox and polio. So we attempt to maintain some level of equilibrium.

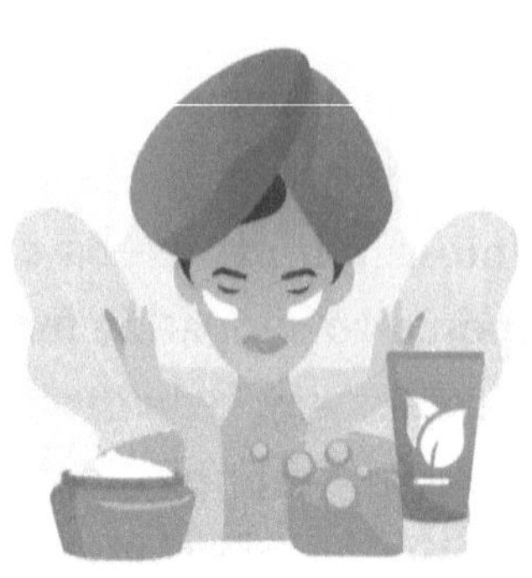

The issue comes when there is a lack of vigilance in adhering to the processes and standards that have been acquired with considerable effort and at tremendous financial and social expense. When it comes to the use of external, topical allopathic medications, there are rigorous criteria and procedures that must be followed when using creams and external preparations. Many people overuse steroid creams. Any skin doctor will tell you horror stories about the overuse and abuse of external applications. Many patients unintentionally overuse steroids, causing harm not just to the skin but also to the metabolic system.

Such problems are never caused by the prudent use of such external drugs. External usage of a basic fairness cream can cause extreme sun sensitivity and accelerate aging changes, but when used sparingly, the same product works wonderfully to give the skin a superb aesthetic look with no adverse effects.

The list of such cases is enormous and might fill many reams of paper. I usually like to use the simile' example to clarify the ideas more thoroughly.

I've often compared the problem of adverse events and side effects in medication to cooking with salt. For example, we don't use salt in sweets in general, so matching the correct drug to a patient's needs is critical; that's what physicians are for, so self-medication is risky.

We must also use the proper amount of salt; prescription dosage is critical, and when properly controlled, it will take care of everything. These principles apply to both allopathic and Ayurvedic therapies.

Also, some people like more salty foods, while others prefer less salty foods, and other people do not require a lot of salt in their diet. Some people abstain from salt as a type of detoxification for their bodies. Similarly, one universal drug will not be enough for each ailment or body type. Furthermore, a basic household component like salt in excess skin treats high blood pressure, and a lack of salt in the elderly can be fatal. Most drugs, such as salt, are safe when administered for the appropriate individual in the correct doses and for the proper durations in both the main systems of allopathy and Ayurveda.

Moving on to numbers 3 and 4, which include the use of botanicals and polyhedral compositions.

Before I address the most prevalent worries regarding heavy metals and harmful substances in herbal remedies, I'd like to bring out some facts.

Fact number one is that many commercially processed food goods include permitted amounts of heavy metals, pesticides, illness causing chemicals, and so on, to the point where numerous samples of a popular ready-to-eat noodles mix were recently at the focus of a large controversy. The debate arose unexpectedly and

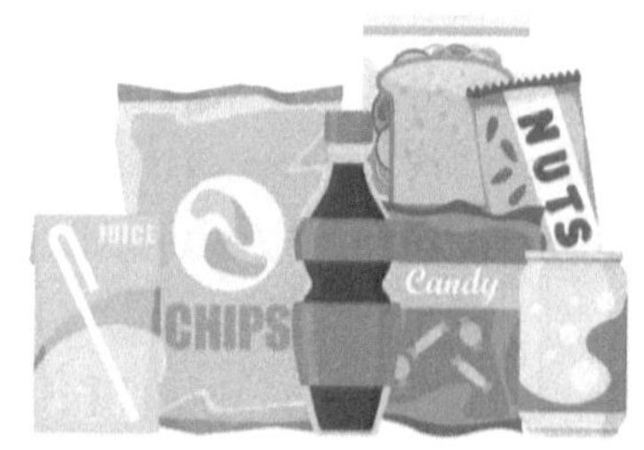

quickly vanished, not just from news outlets but also from our memories.

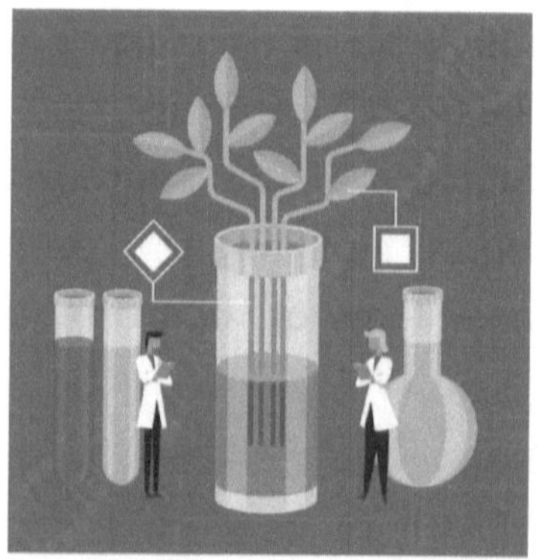

Fact number two is that almost 50 to 60% of popular current allopathic drug systems derive their 'inspiration' from plant origin, and contain chemicals to protect and increase function, absorption of medicines, and so on, which may cause substantial harm. To name a few, several pharmaceuticals, such as Valdecoxib, have been discontinued after selling for billions of dollars, while many others, such as Ranitidine, have been recalled for carrying hazardous ingredients.

The most encouraging aspect of this otherwise depressing data is the existence of a system that appears to be trustworthy and active, deserving of public trust. A mechanism that can evolve and halt the use of such hazardous items once harm caused by them is discovered.

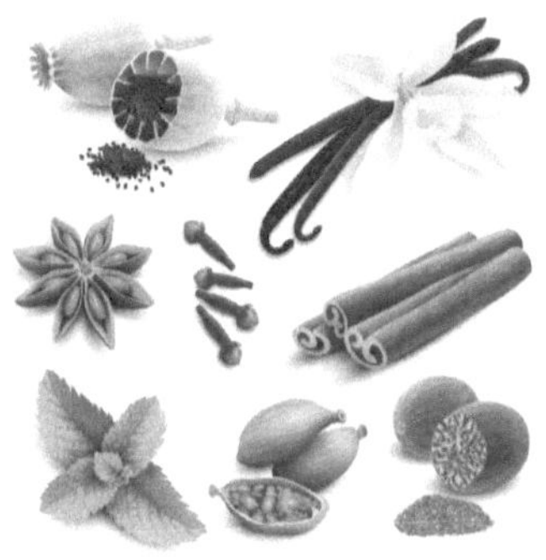

Now that we've gotten into the specifics of some herbs used as medicine, I'd like to mention a few that are commonly used: Amla, liquorice root or mulethi, curry leaves, cinnamon, dhataki flower, saffron, bamboo manna, giloy or Tinospora ordifolia, Tej patta, long pepper or pippali, and many more.

The majority of them are the genuine food supplements that we are discussing. These were typical culinary items in cities as recently as 30-40 years ago, and they remain so in many regions of India and other parts of the world.

Eating bitters to treat a diseased liver is common ethnic knowledge.

To control a suspected parasite infection or to regularize bowel motions, it is usual practice to do a castor oil, senna, or triphala purge.

How dangerous may using their food as medicine be?

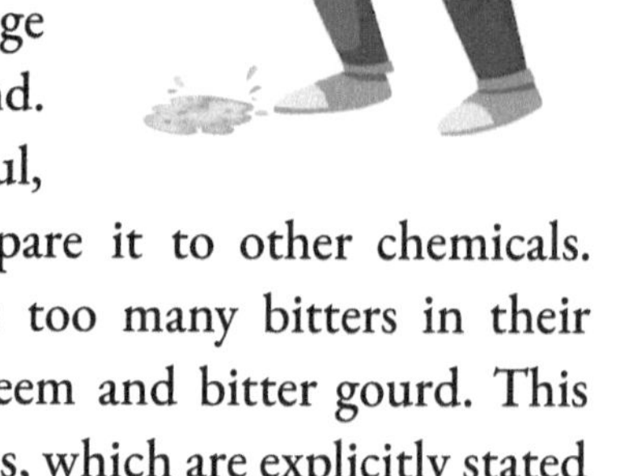

As I mentioned in the salt analogy, I still do not encourage throwing caution to the wind. Food, like salt, can be harmful, but it is impossible to compare it to other chemicals. Again, many individuals use too many bitters in their everyday routines, such as Neem and bitter gourd. This can have negative consequences, which are explicitly stated in ayurveda based on one's body type.

With so much discussion concerning the safety of various herbal formulations, I'd want to add to the hazards that lie when correct dosage is not followed with herbal medication. When adequate production processes are not followed, especially in the case of herbo-mineral or herb-metallic formulations, it can become quite harmful. However, these considerations apply to all parties without exception. Ayurveda should not be held responsible for certain manufacturers breaching the law and getting people sick.

So, to use another comparison, if someone looks at a picture and dislikes it, does the spectator blame the paint or the painter? Ayurveda is the paint, canvas, and tools; how and when they are used defines the product.
Enough 'meal' for thinking has been provided in the preceding sentences.

Now we'll look at how allopathic interventions are used. The similar principle applies to the use of interventional therapies.There are manufacturer rules for machine usage, then there are skills refined through time when any treatment is done for a patient, and there is a long and arduous learning program to skill the physicians, and the risks of errors have been greatly reduced. In general, if someone ignored the rules and procedures, current interventional methods are not to fault.

A simple chemical peel or laser, for example, is certain to produce problems if performed on a patient with inflamed, sensitive, or contraindicated skin. This is not the common foolishness of allopathic medicine.

We are now turning our attention to alternative therapy modalities such as naturopathy and yoga-based detoxes and lifestyle adjustments.

These may involve inducing a therapeutic big bowel purge and inducing vomiting with or without a sinus cavity rinse. You read that correctly. This shatkarma or *shankh prakshalan* idea is an old approach. Massage of therapeutic points on connected or occasionally 'seemingly unrelated' regions may also be included.

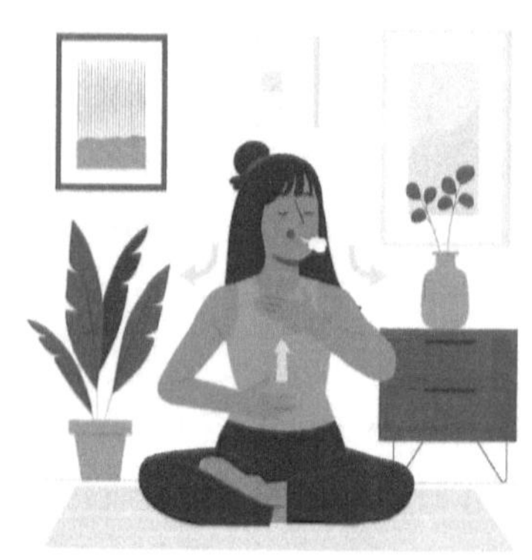

Breathing is also crucial, and basic breathing practices, not pranayama as we know it, are crucial in the delicate balance of health and sickness.To think about it, how much harm can breathing methods cause, especially when taught by a skilled team that has standardized the usage of different techniques for different diseases? How much harm may pressure point marma treatment in the hands of specialists cause you? How much damage may a saltwater or fennel water revocation purge cause? How many negative consequences do they have? How dangerous may a therapeutic method become, even when all safeguards are taken?

I'd like to leave the verdict to our own unique judgments when it comes to determining safety. Once revealed, our genuine inner nature understands what is safe for us.

Even lower animals have protective instincts and avoid eating unhealthy foods. So, because man is such an "intellectual" and superior entity, he will be able to choose what is safe for him.

IS USE OF INTEGRATED DERMATOLOGY MORE EXPENSIVE?

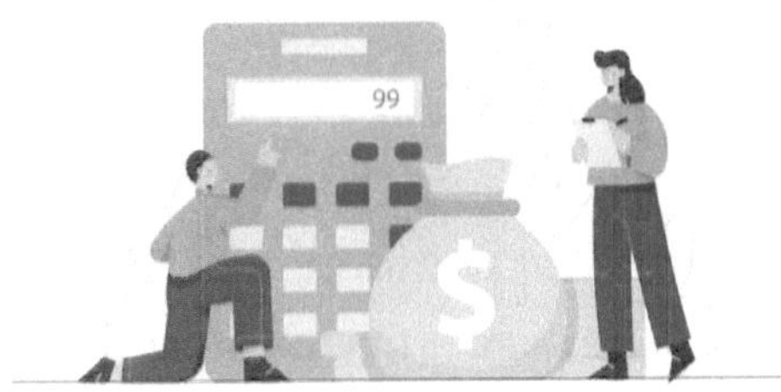

When an integrated review is performed and specialists from several specialties are engaged. Despite the fact that the planning is Handelly.! Allopathic and Ayurvedic specialists To can bond, a medic on a can may be used. This may create the appearance that the carts are higher in a complicated card than in a basic, Pharmacological Subscription bird.....

Fortunately, most people do not require this.

When a joint requires Crosspathy intervention. On a normal long-term loss, it may not be required. The therapy may then be directed solely by your specialty with occasional input from other doctors. The expenses of an integrated medicine consultation can be regarded in terms of the end cost as well as the cost in terms of the work incorporated. The investment of time, effort, and money.... Such a program is well worth it, because the goal is to enhance overall quality of life rather than simply symptoms. The ultimate purpose is to elevate and improve.

Once the primary symptom of the medical condition is under control, other steps are implemented to reduce the pill load and refocus the patient on stimulating the process of auto healing or awakening the person's own power to heal and mend. The fundamental concepts are based on the timeless philosophy of Treating with Nature for 5 Months. The concept is founded on the fundamental principles of yoga, Naturopathy, and Ayurveda.They are such simple philosophies, rather than a paradigm. They are so dimpled that they may be used to treat any sickness that somebody is suffering from. They are relevant to basic illnesses such as cancer metabolic and hormonal abnormalities, which are prevalent and bothersome.

It is everyone's right to awaken after one has healed within. The healer is inside everyone of us, and the simplicity of awakening comes so effortlessly that it is easy to overlook it, to dismiss it.

The awakening that heals It couldn't be pricey, it...... be expensive just like soaking the seer, inhaling air isn't

CHAPTER 2
UNVEILING THE LIMITATIONS OF MODERN MEDICINE

Modern medicine has seen tremendous growth and development, serving as a beacon of hope and advancement in healthcare. Numerous illnesses have been

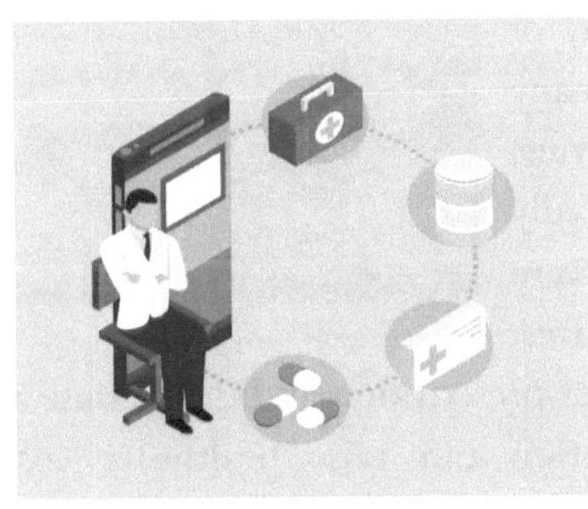

wiped out, lives have been extended, and millions of people's lives have been significantly better. Despite these outstanding accomplishments, modern medicine still has several drawbacks and restrictions. The goal of this study is to critically analyze and illuminate the problems and weaknesses of current therapeutic practice.

1. Concentrate solely on symptom management: Modern medicine's primary focus on managing symptoms rather than treating illnesses' underlying causes is one of its biggest drawbacks. Medications are frequently recommended to address symptoms rather than the underlying problem, offering short-term respite. Although necessary for intense care and quick recovery, this method does not result in lasting recovery or recurrence.

2. Focus too much on treatment and solutions: Drugs are the mainstay of modern medicine for many medical conditions. Drugs have undoubtedly transformed health care and saved countless lives, 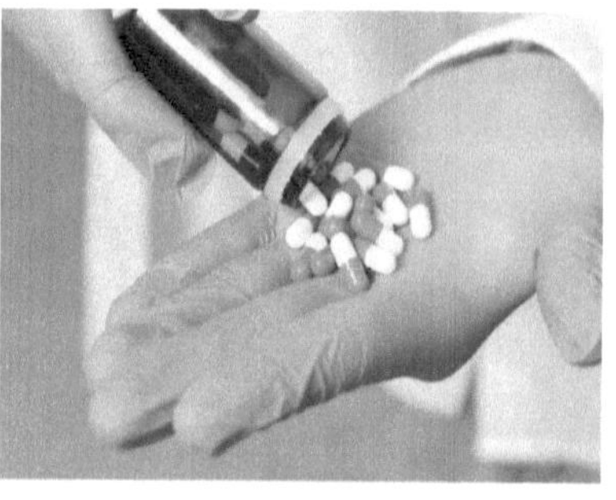 but concerns about over-prescription and drug abuse are growing. Overprescription can raise healthcare costs, expose patients to needless risks, and contribute to antibiotic resistance development.

3. Disease centric approach: Instead of concentrating on a person's entire health and welfare, modern medicine frequently adopts a pathology approach, focusing on certain diseases or ailments. As a result, the healthcare system may become fragmented, with various doctors addressing distinct symptoms or problems in isolation without fully appreciating the patient's overall health.

4. Disparity and difficulty of access: Despite the fact that modern medicine has made enormous advancements, there are still large gaps in access to health care, particularly in developing or economically underdeveloped regions where the high expenses of modern medicine, diagnostic tests, and medications make them unaffordable to the majority of the globe.

5. Findings and problems: There are many adverse effects from modern treatment, including surgery, medication, and therapy. Unwanted side effects, seizures, or other issues that might occasionally be serious or life-threatening may occur in patients. Before deciding whether to utilize a medical intervention, the risks and benefits must be thoroughly considered.

6. Ignoring mental health: In the past, modern medicine frequently disregarded or viewed mental health as a distinct condition from physical health. Despite their ubiquity and importance on general wellbeing, mental health issues have received insufficient attention and inclusion in mainstream medical practice, which has resulted in gaps in total health care due to the relationship between the neglect of mental and physical health. Even when mental health is focused upon, a lot of emphasis is laid on drug management of mental health symptoms, which may result in over medication. The basis for the medication being the theory that there is imbalance of chemical mediators in the neural circuits.

7. Insufficient preventative care: In many instances, modern medicine prioritizes treating illnesses as soon as they manifest rather than emphasizing preventative treatments. Early detection, dietary adjustments, and other preventive health treatments can greatly lower the incidence of illness. These preventative efforts, however, receive little focus or funding.

8. Treating typical ailments: Modern medicine has a propensity to address biological and typical elements, including aging, menstruation, or simple changes in health conditions, and this can result in unneeded, overdiagnosis of medical intervention, overtreatment, and other complications that may be more harmful than helpful.

9. No personalization: In modern medicine, comparable illnesses or ailments are typically treated using standardized protocols in a generalized manner. This universal strategy takes into account the distinctive genetic, environmental, and behavioral elements that influence a person's reaction to therapy. Personalized medicine, in which treatments are tailored to a patient's unique requirements, is a field that is expanding but has not yet entirely permeated daily practice. The newer functional medicine approach to giving personalized advice is expensive as many times it relies on many investigations to find the "root cause" , it relies heavily on the investigation route.

10. Inadequate use of alternative medicine combinations: Although contemporary medicine has made enormous strides, it frequently ignores the potential advantages of complementary and alternative medicine (CAM). CAM can deliver thorough and efficient healthcare when paired with conventional therapies like acupuncture, herbal medicine, and yoga. This integration, nevertheless, is still being developed and is not yet widely recognized.

11. There is disunity in the spiritual component: In favor of concentrating primarily on the physical and, to a lesser extent, psychological components of health, modern medicine routinely ignores the spiritual part of health. Many individuals depend greatly on their faith for their overall well-being because it offers them comfort, purpose, and grit through trying times or when they are ill.

However, medical management does not include the spiritual component, which consists of beliefs, ideals, and practices that foster spiritual welfare.

Neglecting one's spiritual needs: Lack of spiritual integration in medicine ignores the importance of spirituality in holistic healing, illness treatment, and pain control. According to studies, people who have a solid spiritual base frequently use healthy coping mechanisms, experience less stress, and have better results in managing chronic illnesses.

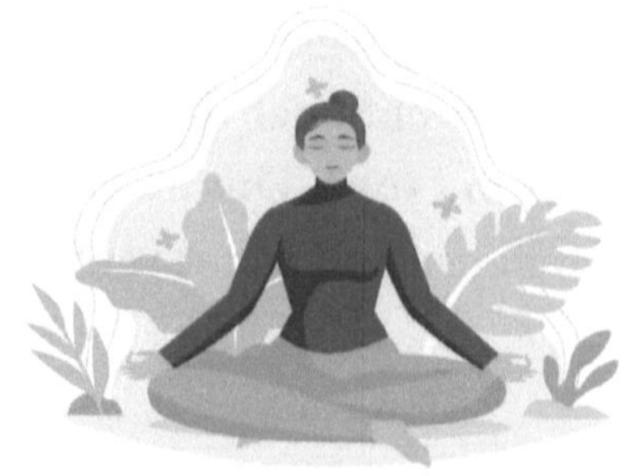

Spiritual health and complementary therapies: Integral to a holistic approach to health is spiritual wellness. Neglecting the spiritual component interferes with patient-centered treatment and a comprehensive perspective of health.

Patient centric approach: The patient experience, adherence to therapies, and general health satisfaction can all be improved by acknowledging and honoring one's spiritual views and incorporating them into the treatment plan. To ensure the most suitable and efficient care, a patient-centered approach should take spiritual views into account.

Resistance to drugs and excellent mental health: Spirituality frequently plays a significant part in fostering adaptability and mental wellness. It provides people with a feeling of meaning, hope, and optimism that can help them manage chronic ailments, get better from illnesses, and cope with difficult life circumstances.

Possible advantages of spiritual union: According to research, including spiritual care into medical treatment can help patients cope with pain better, cope with anxiety and sadness less, and feel better overall. It can also help patients talk about and make decisions about their end-of-life care, giving them support and comfort when they need it most.

A holistic, kind, and patient-centered approach to health treatment can be facilitated by integrating the spiritual component into medicine while respecting faiths and viewpoints. Understanding the significance of spirituality can help people bridge the gap between very personal, spiritual components of their health and healing journeys and medical science.

Conclusion:

Unquestionably, modern medicine has revolutionized healthcare and saved innumerable lives, but it is critical to acknowledge its limitations. A thorough analysis of these restrictions can direct healthcare design in the direction of a thorough, patient-centered, and integrated strategy. By tackling these issues and taking a more holistic approach,

health care can advance toward a time when contemporary medicine's capabilities will be improved and its drawbacks will be lessened, eventually resulting in the benefit of people and communities throughout the world.

CHAPTER 3
UNCOVERING THE LIMITATIONS OF ALTERNATIVE MEDICINE

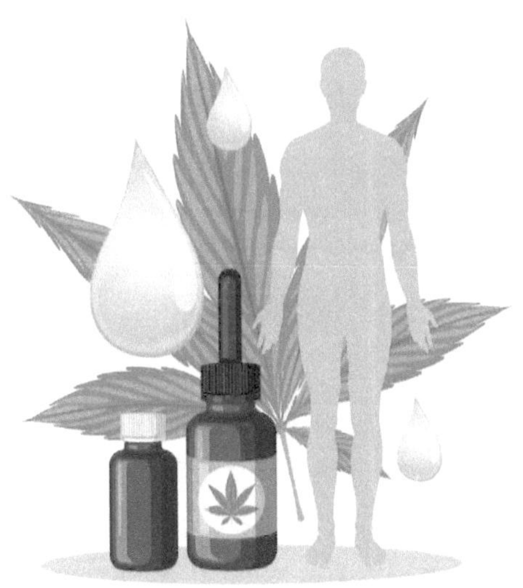

The emerging field of medicine, commonly referred to as complementary alternative medicine (CAM), has gained acceptance and traction in general health and well-being in recent years The study aims to investigate the limitations of drugs as a replacement and clarification.

1. Absence of scientific norms and evidence: The absence of solid scientific data proving alternative medicine's efficacy and safety is one of its main drawbacks. Clinical trials and other rigorous scientific studies are often lacking in novel medicines to support their claims. Without empirical evidence, it becomes challenging to validate the effectiveness and potential risks associated with these treatments. Moreover, the lack of standardized protocols and dosages for many alternative therapies further compounds the issue, making it difficult to replicate results and establish a consistent approach to treatment.

2. Heterogeneity and Fragmentation: Alternative medicine encompasses a vast and heterogeneous array of practices, systems, and therapies, each with its own principles, approaches, and methodologies. This diversity often leads to fragmentation within the field, making it challenging to categorize, regulate, and integrate into mainstream healthcare. The lack of a unified framework can also confuse patients and healthcare professionals, hindering effective communication and collaboration.

3. Delayed or Avoidance of Conventional Medical Treatment: A significant concern is the delay or avoidance of conventional medical treatment by individuals relying solely on alternative therapies. While alternative medicine may offer relief or symptom management, it may not address the underlying cause of a condition or provide life-saving interventions essential in acute or severe health crises. Relying solely on alternative treatments can potentially delay necessary medical care, which can be detrimental, especially in critical situations.

4. Potential harms and consequences: Contrary to the assumption that it is completely safe, alternative therapies can have potential side effects, interactions and complications. For example, herbal supplements can interact with prescription medications, causing side effects or reducing medication effectiveness. Also, some treatments, such as exercise modifications or acupuncture, can cause injuries if done improperly or by practitioners who are not properly trained and understand the harmless natural equations inadequate precautions and monitoring have been taken, resulting in unforeseen health complications. Side effects with such a drug are often difficult to predict, as side effects for the same drug will vary from person to person.

5. Financial costs and lack of insurance: Pursuing alternative treatments can be a financial burden, as many of these treatments are not covered by health insurance plans. These treatments are

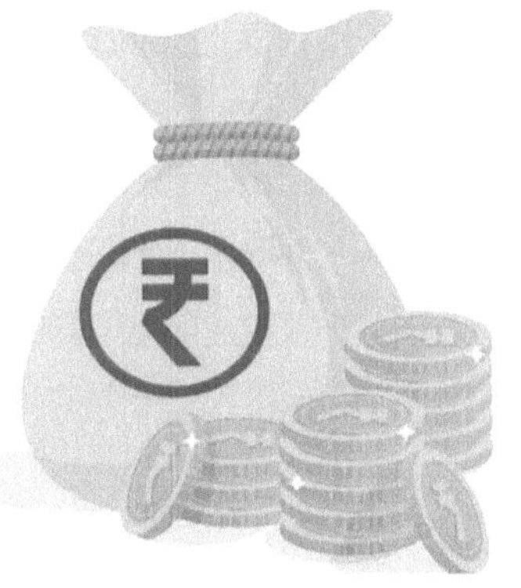

usually paid entirely out of pocket by individuals, making them an expensive endeavor especially with limited financial resources The financial burden can shift or withhold funding from individuals for health care resources, and has severely limited the availability of alternative therapies.

6. Regulatory Challenges and Quality Control: Alternative medicine lacks uniform regulation and oversight compared to conventional medicine. The variability in regulatory standards across countries or regions poses a challenge in ensuring the quality, safety, and efficacy of treatments. Quality control issues, such as contamination of herbal products or inaccuracies in dosages, underscore the need for robust regulation to safeguard the public. There are differences in the way the same medicine is made by different ayurvedic companies, slight differences in methodology or addition or omission of even 1-2 ingredients may play a big role in efficacy and tolerability of medication.for example even a simple amla supplement the way it's made and extracted will have a huge impact of treatment outcomes. If Amla supplement is made by extracting juice in high speed juicers and adding preservatives to it the impact on health may not be as desirable. Same way while preparing amla powder tablets some companies extract co2 extract and some just dry powders, the potency of dry powder will be 5-10 times lesser that co2 extract, but adverse events will also be more with co2 extract.

7. Misinformation and Unrealistic Claims: The proliferation of misinformation and exaggerated claims in the realm of alternative medicine is a significant limitation. The internet and social media platforms can perpetuate misleading information, promoting treatments as 'miracle cures' or 'guaranteed remedies' without scientific substantiation. This misinformation can misguide individuals seeking alternative therapies, potentially causing harm or disappointment when expectations are not met. Many herbal remedies promise cure or control of diabetes, whereas in classical ayurveda it has to be managed a lot by aahar -Vihar which is a lifestyle approach, not just medicines. No medicine can cure poor lifestyle choices.

8. Inadequate Practitioner Training and Credentialing: Certain alternative therapies lack standardized educational requirements and licensing, leading to a disparity in the training and competency of practitioners. Without standardized educational curricula and stringent credentialing, individuals may receive treatments from inadequately trained or unqualified practitioners, risking their safety and the effectiveness of the therapy. This is a commonly seen concern among patients receiving CAM that different physicians have given completely different diagnoses but the same happens in modern medicine also.

9. Conflict with Evidence-Based Medicine: The conflict between alternative medicine and evidence-based medicine, which is grounded in empirical research and proven efficacy, is a significant limitation. In some cases, alternative therapies may contradict established scientific principles or lack empirical validation, creating a divide in the healthcare community. Bridging this gap and fostering collaboration between evidence-based medicine and alternative medicine is essential for a more integrated and informed healthcare approach.

10. Cultural and Ethical Considerations: Alternative medicine often draws from traditional or cultural practices deeply rooted in specific communities. While these practices may have cultural significance, they may not align with modern medical and ethical standards. Balancing cultural appreciation with safety, efficacy, and informed consent becomes a challenge, emphasizing the need for critical evaluation and cultural competence in providing alternative therapies.

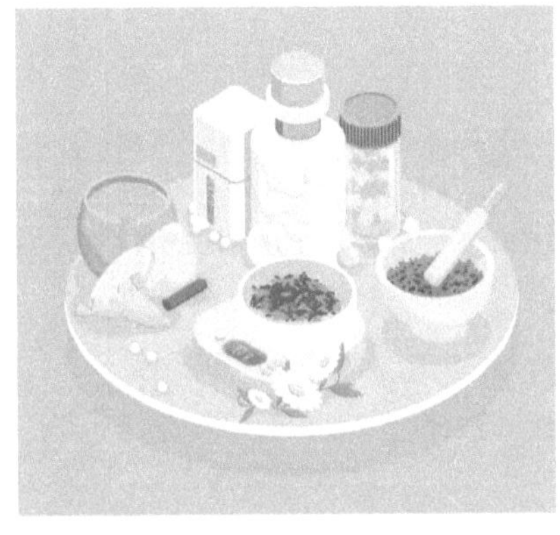

11. Poly herbal formulations pose a challenge to use predictably: Many times there are more than 1 herbs, or ingredients in the herbal medication, making it tough to predict effects and side effects and completely and comprehensively understand the way it will be moving and metabolizing in the body. There are some commonly used ayurvedic formulations containing more than 40 individual herbs and extracts. In such cases the safety and predictability becomes next to impossible. Also when it comes to polyherbal preparations, many times if some ingredient is unavailable due to any reason, the companies may formulate with what is available due to market forces. This can impact efficacy and treatment, also there does not exist a mechanism to detect such practices once the product hits the shelves.

> **TIP -CASE OF OVER USED HERBAL PRODUCTS CAUSING TROUBLE**
>
> *A patient was prescribed digestive ayurvedic preparation for a period of 20 days and along with that few dietary changes and recommendation to sleep on time and chew food well. The patient experienced good improvement in symptoms and on his own kept taking the "digestive ayurvedic pills" without following much of the other recommendations for a period of 3 months. This led to a serious life threatening bout of gastric ulcers, which not only were expensive to treat but also led to unnecessary morbidity.*

Conclusion

Alternative medicine holds the promise of providing holistic and personalized healthcare, which meets the preferences of many individuals in both natural and non-invasive treatments but is necessary if we recognize and accept limitations in this diverse and growing field acknowledge.Clinicians, academics, politicians, and the general public must work together to ensure that alternatives are properly and successfully incorporated into the healthcare system in order to overcome these restrictions. We may work toward a knowledgeable and well-balanced approach to health and wellness that incorporates the qualities of conventional and alternative medicine by improving rigorous research, standards, regulation, and education.

CHAPTER 4
HEALING THE WHOLE YOU: WHY INTEGRATIVE MEDICINE MATTERS

General approach Medicine, at its core, is concerned with treating and restoring health. Various medical systems have emerged throughout history, each offering unique methods for achieving this goal. Both integrative and applied medicine represent a modern response to the limitations and challenges posed by traditional medical models.

In this talk, we will explore the critical importance of integrated and holistic medicine—physically, mentally, and emotionally—by treating the whole person and building their potential as health care emphasis will be changed.

Limitations of Traditional Medicine

Traditional Western medicine, commonly referred to as allopathic medicine, tends to focus on the management of symptoms and the treatment of disease with drugs, surgery, and other methods. There are some limitations:

Reductionist Approach: Traditional medicine generally takes a reductionist approach, dividing the human body into separate systems and treating each separately This can give the body of the functions not related to each other.

Focus on symptoms: The first step is symptom monitoring and diagnosis based on specific criteria. Although important, this narrow view may overlook the causes or effects.

Too much emphasis on medicine: The pharmaceutical industry plays an important role in traditional medicine. While medications can save lives, they can lead to over-dependence, side effects and obscure underlying issues. At the cost of sounding repetitive or the risk of being called a plagiarist, I would like to repeat the lines of Dr. B.M

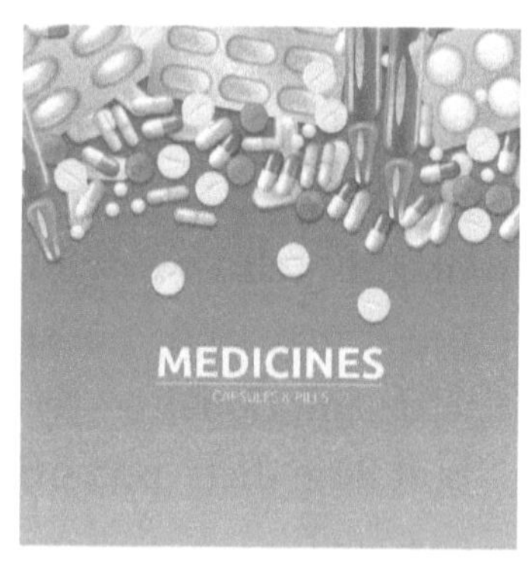

Hegde that " There does not exist a pill for every ill , but there is an ill after every pill"

Ignoring mental and emotional well-being: Mental health is often treated separately from physical health, leading to a misunderstanding of a person's overall well-being

Emergence of Integrative Holistic Medicine

In response to these limitations, integrative holistic medicine has developed. These approaches aim to address the gaps by considering the whole person, lifestyle, and underlying factors that affect health. Here's why it matters:

Treating the whole person: Integrative and holistic medicine views the person as a complex system in which mind, body and spirit are interconnected and interdependent. By considering all aspects of a person's life—physical, emotional, social, environmental, and spiritual—these strategies address the root causes of health issues rather than reducing them just by symptoms.

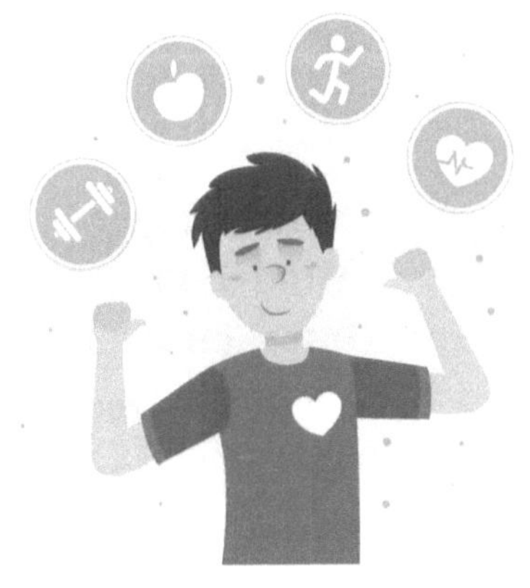

Focus on disease prevention and health promotion: One of the basic principles of all combination therapy is disease prevention. Rather than waiting for diseases to appear, these strategies emphasize preventive measures such as healthy eating, regular exercise, stress reduction, and a balanced lifestyle. By doing this , this quality priority reduces the incidence of disease and contributes to quality of life.

Integration of alternative traditional medicine: Integrative medicine combines the best of traditional and complementary medicine. It recognizes the advances and benefits of traditional therapies and incorporates alternative evidence-based therapies such as acupuncture, chiropractic, herbal medicine, mindfulness practices, etc. This combination provides a comprehensive and personalized approach as they use treatment.

Patient empowerment: A holistic and integrated approach to healthcare that actively involves the patient in their healing journey. Patients are encouraged to actively participate in their healthcare decision-making, and given a sense of power and accountability. This collaborative approach often leads to better management of treatments and improved outcomes.

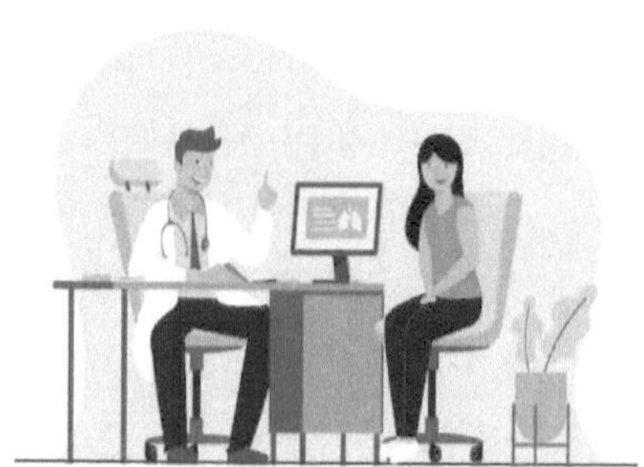

Addressing the Mind-Body Interaction: Holistic practice recognizes the undeniable connection between mental and physical health. Stress, anxiety, and emotional trauma can manifest physically. Holistic medicine achieves more intensive treatment by addressing emotional and mental wellbeing through techniques such as meditation, yoga and mindfulness therapy.

Individual treatment plans: Everyone is different, what works for one may not work for another. The integration of holistic approaches can lead to treatment programs tailored to each individual's unique needs, preferences, and circumstances. This individualization often produces effective and lasting results.

Conclusion

The need for comprehensive and inclusive health care is more important than ever in a world with a wide range of complicated health concerns. Traditional medical models have holes that integrative and holistic medicine fills to produce a revolutionary approach that cares for the full individual. By adopting these tactics, we're laying the groundwork for a healthier future where people are empowered to actively manage their health and attain their ideal levels of fitness and health. Traditional supplementary medicine is building the framework for a new age in healthcare—one that prioritizes holistic treatment and improves everyone's quality of life—by emphasizing illness prevention and the mind-body link. Integrative and holistic approach is the true embodiment of the P4I medicine concept of participative, preventive, predictive personalized and integrated medicine approach. Which we elaborate more in the next chapter.

CHAPTER 5
P4 medicine

Integrative Dermatology is naturally founded on P4 -predictive, preventative, personalized, participatory medicine.The notion of P4 medicine has greatly altered the approach to healthcare in recent years. P4 medicine, which stands for Predictive, Preventive, Personalized, and Participatory medicine, is strongly related to integrated dermatological ideas.

PREDICTIVE:
P4 medicine focuses on health and illness prediction. It entails the use of modern diagnostic techniques, genetic profiling, and other cutting-edge technology to identify possible risks and predict the occurrence of certain skin disorders. Predictive factors in integrated dermatology enable for early intervention and proactive actions to preserve skin health.

PREVENTIVE:
Prevention is central to both P4 medicine and integrative dermatology. The emphasis changes to preventative methods when dangers are identified early by using prediction technologies. Patients are taught on lifestyle changes, skincare regimens, and environmental variables that can prevent skin disorders from forming or worsening.

PERSONALIZED:

P4 Medicine and Integrative Dermatology both value tailored care. They understand that because each person is unique, one method will not suffice. The formulation of treatment programs based on an individual's particular genetics, lifestyle, preferences, and skin profile is known as personalization. This method enhances treatment results while also increasing patient satisfaction and adherence to the treatment plan.

PARTICIPATORY:

Active patient engagement is another critical component of combining P4 therapy with dermatology. Patients are urged to take an active role in their health care, understand their skin, and collaborate with their healthcare team in order to make sound decisions. Skin integration allows patients to participate in their treatment plan, make lifestyle changes, and take prescription medications as indicated.

For example, a busy executive with a lot of travel 2-3 times per month, was struggling to incorporate fasting in their routine. A simple discussion about their travel plans, nature of travel was done and a recommendation was mutually agreed upon to make small, simply doable tweaks in meal time so that long hours of 18-24 hours of intermittent or water only fast can be incorporated during travel time and sleep time. This really helped in not only reducing exposure to eating out, but enhanced metabolic health, performance at work, sleep quality and energy levels of the patient. It is now a regular practice with him during his frequent travels. Understanding your body is the key to health.

Incorporating Principles of P4 Medicine into Dermatological Practice

Integrative dermatologists apply P4 medicine ideas in the following ways:

Utilizing Genetic Insights: Integrative dermatologists may use genetic testing to better understand a patient's susceptibility to particular skin disorders. This data is used to develop individualized treatment programs and prevention tactics.

Educating for Prevention: Integrative dermatologists teach patients about lifestyle changes, sun protection, and skincare regimens to avoid skin disorders and preserve good skin by using predictive and preventative techniques.

Tailoring Treatment Plans: Integrative dermatologists apply P4 principles to personalize treatment programs to each patient's individual needs, taking genetic variables, medical history, lifestyle, and environmental effects into account.

Patient Engagement: Integrative dermatology promotes active patient engagement in order to ensure that patients are well-informed, engaged, and dedicated to their skin health journey.

The incorporation of P4 medicine ideas into integrative dermatology is a game-changing approach to skin health. This strategy aims to change dermatological care by forecasting risks, concentrating on prevention, tailoring treatments, and encouraging active patient engagement, ultimately resulting in better results and a higher quality of life for individuals.

"Case of severe recurring acne managed with custom lifestyle changes"

A 26 Year old female patient was having acne despite courses of oral isotretinoin, antibiotics and some hormonal treatments. There was a regular breakout of cystic and papulo-pustular acne especially pre periods. All investigations were normal, ultrasounds and other investigations for hormone evaluation.

She was managed with oral anti inflammatory enzymes, 4gm/ day of inositol supplements. Some herbs were added as per her body type, like coriander, mint, fennel in higher quantities. Dairy and processed food was stopped for 20 days. There was not only remarkable improvement but with each cycle the severity of acne reduced. Once she developed a deeper understanding of dietary choices aggravating acne, she became more aware and connected with her food. The patient assessment at the end of 3 months was a superior improvement in skin quality , acne outbreaks and quality of life, digestion, and sleep as compared to conventional treatment, which was playing with her mood. Isotretinoin and synthetic oral contraceptive pills are known to have a host of adverse effects.

CHAPTER 6
EVIDENCE OF YOGA AND NATUROPATHY-BASED TREATMENTS

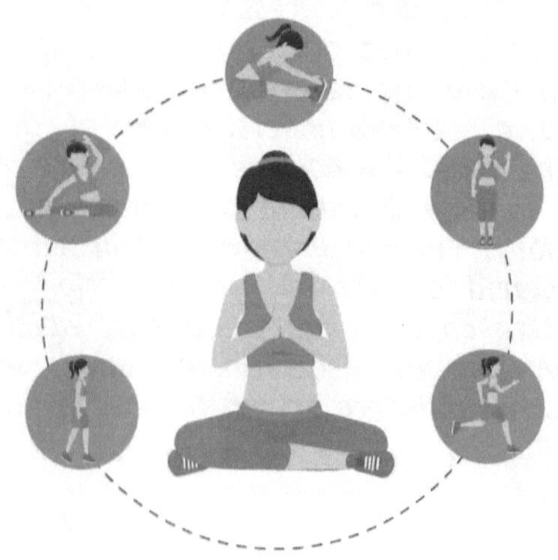

Modern times have seen a huge increase in the popularity of yoga and naturopathy, two traditional holistic healthcare systems that have a long history of treating a variety of illnesses. Despite having a long history, these behaviors are the subject of current scientific research. In-depth analysis of the substantial research demonstrating yoga and naturopathy positive effects on both physical and mental health is presented in this chapter.

Yoga-based therapies

Yoga, which has its roots in ancient India, is a comprehensive wellness regimen that includes breathing exercises (pranayama), meditation, and moral principles in addition to physical postures (asanas). Over time, thorough scientific investigation has produced convincing proof of yoga's numerous advantages, making it a crucial supplement to medical procedures.

Benefits for Physical Health

1. Management of chronic pain:

Yoga appears to be a good treatment for managing chronic pain, including migraines, arthritis, and lower back pain. According to research in JAMA Internal Medicine, yoga dramatically reduced persistent low back pain when compared to standard medical treatment.

2. Strength and flexibility are improved:

Regular yoga practice improves both muscle strength and flexibility. According to a review in Complementary Therapies in Medicine, yoga significantly improves musculoskeletal problems and lowers the chance of injury.

3. Heart and Vascular Health:

Through its ability to lower blood pressure, cholesterol levels, and the risk of heart disease, yoga has a favorable impact on cardiovascular health. Yoga has the potential to enhance cardiovascular fitness overall and heart health, according to the European Journal of Preventive Cardiology.

Benefits for Mental Health

1. Reduced Stress:

Yoga stands out as a powerful stress-reduction method. According to research in the Journal of Clinical Oncology, yoga dramatically lowers stress levels and improves quality of life for those with breast cancer.

2. Management of Depression and Anxiety:

According to research, yoga can be quite helpful in treating anxiety and depression. According to a meta-analysis that was published in JAMA Psychiatry, yoga was linked to a mild reduction in depression symptoms.

3. Enhanced Cognitive Performance:

Regular yoga practice has been associated with enhanced memory and cognitive performance. A research in the Journal of Physical Activity and Health highlighted the benefits of yoga on older individuals' cognitive function.

4.Improved standard of living

The benefits of yoga go beyond the worlds of the body and mind. According to research that was published in the International Journal of Yoga Therapy, yoga treatments dramatically increased the quality of life for people with different chronic diseases.

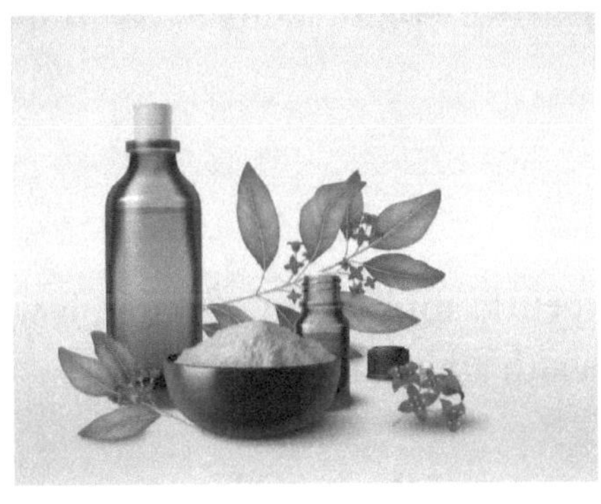

Treatments Based on Naturopathy

Naturopathy depends on organic treatments, dietary changes, and the body's natural ability to heal itself. It focuses a strong emphasis on giving the body the tools it needs to restore balance and encourage self-healing using the resources of nature.

Nutrition and Diet

1. Managing Chronic Illnesses:

Dietary management of chronic disorders like diabetes and hypertension is supported by research. Dietary treatments are crucial for managing diabetes, according to research published in the Journal of Diabetes Research.

2. Weight Control:

In naturopathy, keeping a healthy weight is based on a balanced food and way of life. The International Journal of Obesity published a comprehensive review that showed how successful naturopathic weight control techniques are.

Hydrotherapy

Hydrotherapy, the therapeutic application of water, is well known for its range of health advantages.

1. Pain relief and relaxation of the muscles

Hydrotherapy has shown potential in reducing pain and relaxing muscles. The benefits of hydrotherapy in treating pain were emphasized in a research that was published in the Journal of Advanced Nursing.

2. Better Circulation

Blood circulation is reported to be improved by hydrotherapy. A study that appeared in the Journal of Clinical Medicine Research showed how hydrotherapy enhanced peripheral circulation.

Herbal remedies

Herbal medicine is commonly used in naturopathy to treat a variety of diseases.

1. Treatment of Digestive Conditions:

Digestive issues can be effectively treated using herbal treatments. The potential of herbal medicines in treating gastrointestinal problems was covered in a review published in the World Journal of Gastroenterology.

2. Pain Control:

The control of pain can be effectively accomplished with certain herbal remedies. The analgesic properties of herbal treatments were highlighted by a study published in Evidence-Based Complementary and Alternative Medicine.

Conclusion

The search discussed in this chapter highlights the yoga and naturopathy-based therapies' enormous potential to improve both physical and mental health. However, it is critical to recognize that each patient's reaction to these treatments may differ, underscoring the significance of a customized strategy. Following an evidence-based methodology, incorporating yoga and naturopathy into healthcare procedures promotes a more holistic approach to healthcare, improving general well-being and quality of life.

It's crucial to remember that this summary only offers a broad picture of the data; for a complete understanding, a careful reading of particular studies and research articles is advised. As usual, seeking advice from a healthcare expert is advised before beginning any new therapy or treatment. We'll examine specific case studies and delve into the real-world implementations of these holistic healthcare systems in the chapters that follow.

CHAPTER 7:
NEED FOR SPIRITUAL QUOTIENT IN TREATING DISEASES

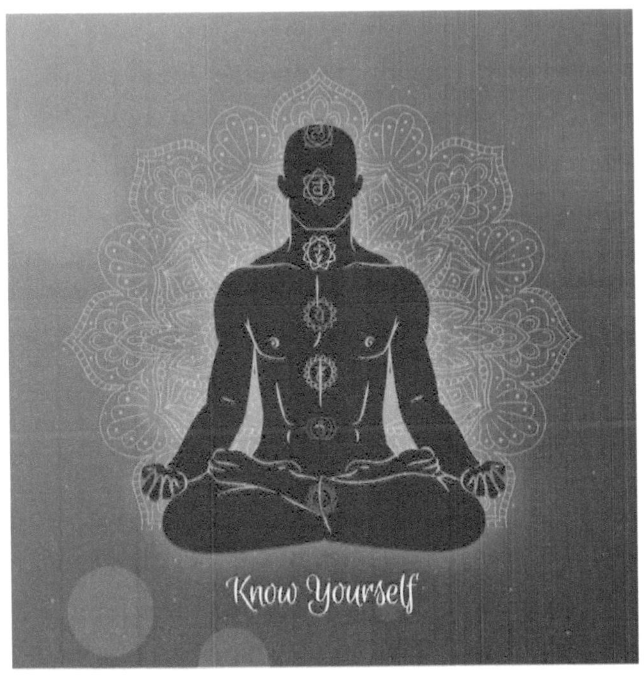

This chapter's expanded review explores the urgent necessity to incorporate spiritual quotient (SQ) into the field of disease therapy. This chapter provides a thorough grasp of the importance of spirituality in healthcare, supported by references and extra resources.

It is undeniable that modern medicine has made significant strides in treating a variety of disorders. However, it has mostly concentrated on the physical components of health, frequently ignoring the complex interactions between a person's physical, mental, emotional, and spiritual dimensions.This chapter examines the growing acceptance and integration of spirituality as a necessary component for reaching a more holistic approach to healing, as assessed by the concept of "spiritual quotient" (SQ).

What is Spiritual Quotient ?

Similar to emotional quotient (EQ) and intelligence quotient (IQ), spiritual quotient (SQ) is a relatively new notion. It aims to gauge a person's spiritual understanding and intelligence. SQ includes traits like *the **ability to find meaning and purpose in life*** as well as traits like empathy, compassion, inner serenity, and resilience. In order to achieve holistic wellbeing, one must also have the capacity to communicate with one's inner self, other people, nature, and the divine.

Spirituality and Health

1. Psychosomatic Relationship:

There is a strong and complex link between spirituality and health. According to scientific research, spiritual beliefs and practices may have an impact on stress levels, immunological function, and the neuroendocrine system. This connection demonstrates how strongly physical health and spiritual well-being influence one another. (1)

2. Resilience and Stress Reduction:

It has been demonstrated that spiritual practices including mindfulness, meditation, and prayer increase resilience and lower stress levels. These techniques foster inner tranquility, enhanced coping skills, and a more upbeat approach, all of which are essential for managing chronic illnesses and accelerating recovery.(2)

Role of Spirituality in Disease Management

1. Chronic Illnesses:

The importance of spirituality in treating chronic illnesses is growing. It has been demonstrated that incorporating spirituality into treatment programs can help pain management in conditions including cancer, heart disease,

and diabetes, as well as improve patients' quality of life.
(3)

2. Mental health conditions:

Growing evidence suggests that spirituality may have therapeutic benefits for mental health. It has shown promise to use spiritual practices to address issues including addiction, anxiety, and depression. (4)

Holistic Healing Methods

1. Patient holistic care:

A holistic approach takes into account a person's physical, mental, emotional, and spiritual well-being as a whole. Spirituality is incorporated into patient care to create a more thorough and individualized approach that promotes healing on many levels.(5)

2. End-of-Life Care:

In palliative and end-of-life care, spirituality is crucial in assisting patients and their families to find comfort, acceptance, and purpose during trying times. For a peaceful transition and the best possible quality of life in their final stages, those who are approaching death must have their spiritual needs met.(6)

Issues and Moral Considerations

1. Cultural Awareness:

Integrating spirituality into healthcare can be difficult due to the diversity of cultural and religious views that must be understood and respected. Healthcare practitioners must address this matter delicately, ensuring that spiritual treatment is suitable for local cultures.([7])

2. Aware Consent and Independence:

It is crucial to respect the autonomy and beliefs of patients. In order to guarantee that patients are at ease and that their preferences are honored, it is crucial to gain their informed consent before incorporating spiritual elements into the treatment plan.([8])

Conclusion

A more thorough and effective way to treat diseases depends on recognizing and incorporating spirituality into medical procedures. A person's wellbeing, resiliency, and capacity to handle different health issues can be significantly impacted by their level of spirituality. Healthcare practitioners and systems need to accept spirituality and include it into treatment plans in order to provide a thorough and patient-centered healing process. Improvements in patient outcomes and general satisfaction with healthcare experiences will surely result from this strategy.

Case: stress induced urticaria and a case of stress induced Acne rosacea.

This is about 2 patients, both 25 and 35 yr old females who had these concerns of stress induced urticaria and stress induced rosacea flares. There were almost daily flares of intensely red itchy urticaria wheals and flares wherever there was an apparent stressful situation or there was intense fast paced activity like getting late for a meeting or a meeting presentation at office etc. intense arguments and heated debates with family and friends were also a cause for trigger.

Along with all the standard symptomatic and supportive treatments for urticaria and rosacea the patients were encouraged to listen to lectures and discourses on vedanta concept of advaita and the "concept of being the witness" -Sakshi bhava. The patients were instructed to listen to audio lectures every day for 30 minutes daily about the specific topics during their commute time or free time. They were also encouraged to contemplate about this by sitting in silence for 10-15 minutes before bed time daily. Within 3 weeks the patients reported being less reactive during similar stress triggering situations and both of them reported significantly reduced symptom flares. By the end of 3 months the need for symptomatic treatments like anti allergics, anxiolytics and topical anti redness products for rosacea went down significantly.
There were symptom aggravations occasionally but once the patients became more aware and connected to the root causes they were able to manage their symptoms without any oral medication.

CHAPTER 8
Integrated V/s Integrative Dermatology

The diagnosis, treatment, and management of skin-related issues are the focus of the constantly developing field of dermatology. Integrated Dermatology and Integrative Dermatology are two separate systems that have developed over time, each with its own specific philosophy and methodologies. In this chapter, we'll set out on a quest to comprehend the fundamental distinctions and affinities between these two schools of thought, shedding light on how these two schools have shaped the field of contemporary dermatological care.

A Unified Approach to Integrated Dermatology

A skin care paradigm called integrated dermatology unites various medical disciplines under one roof to create a seamless and well-coordinated solution to dermatological problems. In this method, dermatologists work closely with other medical specialists like general practitioners, surgeons, and pathologists. Patients with a range of skin disorders can benefit from a thorough assessment and treatment plan thanks to our collaboration. The foundation of integrated dermatology is the idea that effective treatment is best provided when a group of specialists collaborate and share their knowledge.

Integrative dermatology is concerned with:

1. **Efficiency:** By removing the need for referrals and several appointments, patients can gain from quicker and more direct access to specialized care.

2. **Multidisciplinary expertise:** Bringing together the abilities and expertise of several professionals improves the accuracy of diagnoses and the efficacy of treatments.

3. **Patient Experience is Simplified:** Patients frequently find the integrated approach more convenient because all of their healthcare needs are fulfilled in one place.

4. **Evidence-Based Practices:** Integrated Dermatology bases its patient care on the most recent findings in science.

A holistic approach to integrative dermatology

Integrative dermatology is a comprehensive approach to skin health that combines complementary therapies with the best methods of traditional dermatology. With this strategy, dermatologists add methods and therapies from conventional and alternative medicine to their toolbox. Integrative dermatology bases its practice on the idea that treating skin problems at their source is essential to a patient's overall health and wellbeing. This method recognises that occasionally the solution to skin health may lie outside the realm of traditional medicine.

Integrative dermatology has a focus on:

1. Holistic well-being: Patients are urged to think about their holistic well-being, which includes lifestyle, stress, and diet as elements that affect the condition of their skin.

2. Complementary Therapies: Dermatologists may advise patients to use complementary therapies like acupuncture, herbal remedies, and mind-body exercises.

3. Personalized Care: Integrative Dermatology creates treatment regimens that are specific to each patient's requirements, taking into account not just their skin issues but also their mental and emotional health.

4. Root Cause Exploration: Rather than only treating symptoms, this strategy aims to find and address the underlying reasons of skin problems.

Here are a few examples about the root cause approach.

Example 1- For a patient of recurring seborrheic dermatitis or severe dandruff, a doctor with functional or integrative approach will not consider the role of fungus/yeast growth as the real cause, rather that is an outcome of something which is allowing to fungus to overgrow on the skin. We would rather look at what are the possible causes leading up to yeast build up on the skin and the body reacting to it which is causing the outcome of seborrheic dermatitis.

Example 2 - The concern of Acne or pimples- The root cause is not the blockage of sebaceous glands nor is the root cause of acne the acne causing bacteria. These are outcomes of single or multiple factors which led to the blocking of oil glands and change in the quality of oil and infection setting in. The approach will be to look for a target for those factors in the individual which are making the sebaceous glands more prone to blocking and infection causing acne.

Example: Psoriasis or other inflammatory skin diseases These diseases too are considered to be an outcome rather than the actual diagnosis alone. An approach to reducing all factors that aggravate inflammation goes a long way in reducing the medicine burden on patients and reducing disease severity. For example, for some patients improving sleep quality and quantity significantly reduces disease symptoms.

A Closer Look at Integrated vs. Integrative Dermatology

While Integrative Dermatology and Integrated Dermatology may seem to be separate disciplines, they are not antagonistic. These methods may work well together to give patients a thorough and all-encompassing approach to skin health.

To give patients a more comprehensive experience, Integrated Dermatology may occasionally integrate integrative components by collaborating with holistic practitioners. On the other hand, when necessary, integrative dermatology may use traditional medical procedures.

A distinction often used in terms, technically, is that Integrated dermatology will provide holistic care within 1 center or 1 person or 1 point of contact who is trained in both tradition and modern dermatological methods. Specialist or super specialists opinions can be sought from time to time. whereas in integrative dermatological care there are more than 1 decision makers, the patient is

taking opinions of modern and traditional opinions separately and a joint discussion or protocol guides to holistic care. Integrative is more of an approach to patient care with best interests in mind.

It's crucial to keep in mind that both strategies aim to give patients the greatest possible treatment for their skin health. The dermatological community increasingly recognizes the advantages of mixing parts from both techniques, eventually helping the patient, as opposed to seeing them as competing forces.

With a clear knowledge of the fundamental distinctions and interactions between Integrated and Integrative Dermatology, we can set out on an exploration of their varied uses to improve patient care and promote skin health.

PART 2: UNDERSTANDING AND MANAGING DERMATOLOGICAL CONDITIONS

CHAPTER 9
ACNE

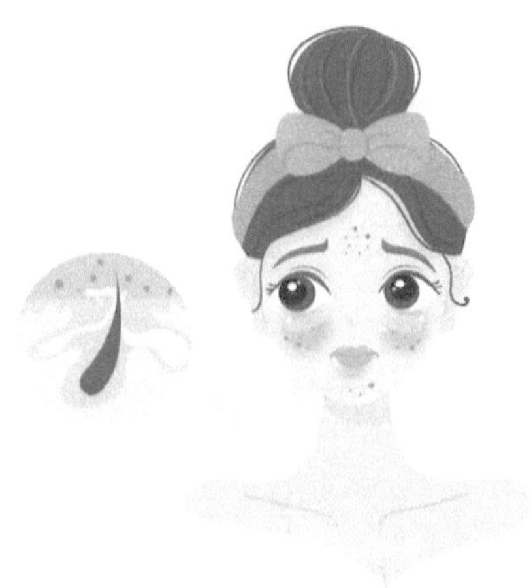

Causes of acne according to allopathy

Commonly referred to as acne, acne vulgaris is a widespread skin condition that mostly affects teenagers and young adults. Its effects on people go well beyond the surface, influencing their quality of life and sense of self-worth. Acne vulgaris is a disorder with several causes that is best understood in the context of allopathy, or mainstream medicine's approach to health. In this chapter, we explore the intricate pathophysiology and identify the key actors responsible for this skin condition.

Abnormal Sebum Production:

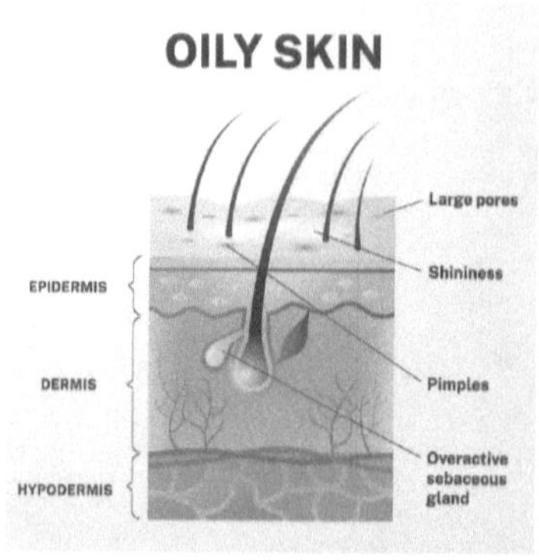

The secretion of excessive amounts of sebum, an oily material produced normally by the sebaceous glands, is the primary cause of acne development. Sebum is essential for lubricating the skin and maintaining its health and vibrancy.

However, excessive sebum production can set off a series of unfavorable events that result in follicular clogging and the development of comedones, those microscopic but bothersome lumps that are associated with acne.(9)

Bacterial Overgrowth (Propionibacterium acnes)

On human skin, there is a bacteria known as Propionibacterium acnes, or P. acnes for short. But when it comes to acne, it grows out of control inside hair follicles. By releasing inflammatory mediators, this overgrowth

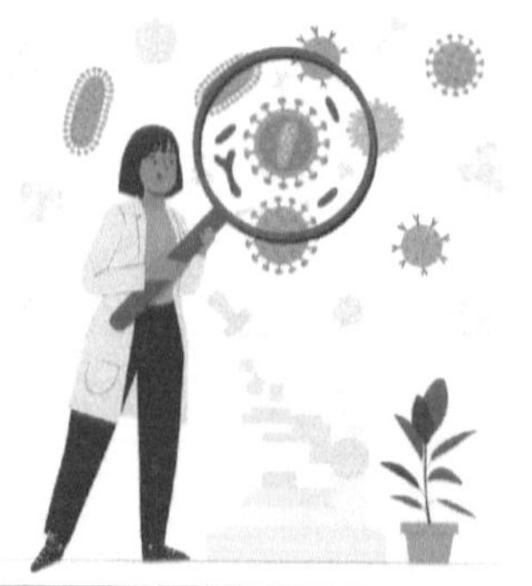

initiates inflammation and contributes to the redness and swelling that characterize acne lesions. (10)

Hyperkeratinization of the follicles:

The complex pathophysiology of acne includes follicular hyperkeratinization as a major role. The abnormal buildup of keratin within hair follicles is referred to by this name. The result is the growth of comedones as a result of the blockage of the pilosebaceous unit, the intricate union of a hair follicle and a sebaceous gland that may serve as an acne-breeding ground.(11)

Changing Hormonal Levels:

The fluctuating hormones, especially the increase in androgens throughout puberty, act as a trigger and aggravating factor for acne. Androgens, often known as male hormones, cause sebaceous glands to create more sebum and have an impact on the maturation of follicular epithelial cells, which promotes the growth of acne.(12)

Irritation:

It is impossible to overestimate the significance of inflammation in the etiology of acne. Microcomedones, a precursor to more problematic acne lesions, appear at the start of the process. The occurrence of this causes the release of cytokines, chemokines, and immune cells, which results in an inflammatory reaction. This reaction results in the formation of the red, uncomfortable, and swollen acne lesions that are frequently referred to as "inflammatory acne."(13)

Lifestyle and Dietary Factors:

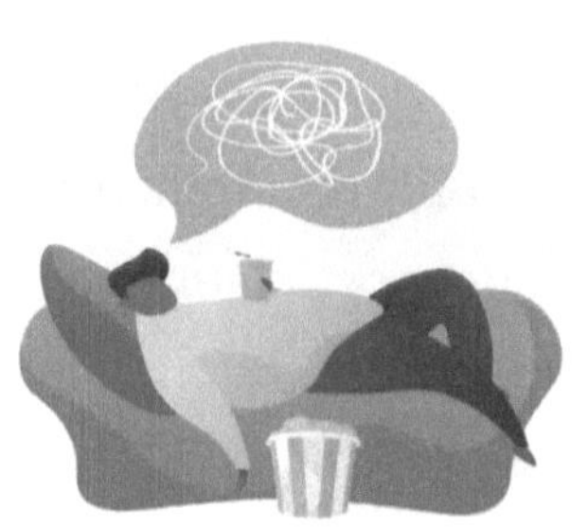

Even while the connection between nutrition and acne is still under investigation, certain studies suggest fascinating correlations. These studies demonstrate a connection between dairy intake, high-glycemic-index diets, and the development of acne. The hormonal balance can also be affected by lifestyle factors, particularly stress, which may exacerbate acne.(14)

Genetic Propensity:

Acne susceptibility is significantly influenced by a person's genetic makeup. According to studies, children who have two parents with a history of acne are more likely to struggle with the condition.(15)

Environmental aspects:

Our living conditions can have a big impact on how bad our acne gets. Acne symptoms might get worse due to things like pollution exposure and excessive humidity levels. Additionally, several chemicals or oils that are often used in a variety of professions might function as triggers in those with acne predispositions.(16)

For the purpose of developing efficient treatment regimens, it is crucial to comprehend these complex causes of acne. To control and lessen the effects of acne vulgaris, allopathic therapies frequently include topical drugs, oral medicines, and lifestyle modifications. Furthermore, continuing studies continue to deepen our understanding of the complexity relating to this widespread yet puzzling skin disorder.

Causes of Acne According to Ayurveda

The traditional medical system of ancient India known as Ayurveda provides a distinctive viewpoint on the reasons why people get pimples, also known as "Yuvan Pidika" or "Mukha Dushika." According to Ayurveda, acne and pimples are a reflection of physiological and psychological as well as lifestyle-related imbalances inside the body. In order to treat acne holistically in Ayurveda, it is crucial to comprehend these factors.

The Dosha Imbalance

The idea of doshas, the underlying forces that control our bodies, is a cornerstone of ayurveda. Acne is frequently linked to an imbalance in the Pitta dosha, which stands for the components of fire and water. Pitta excess can cause the body to become overheated, which can cause skin breakouts and inflammation.

Inappropriate diet

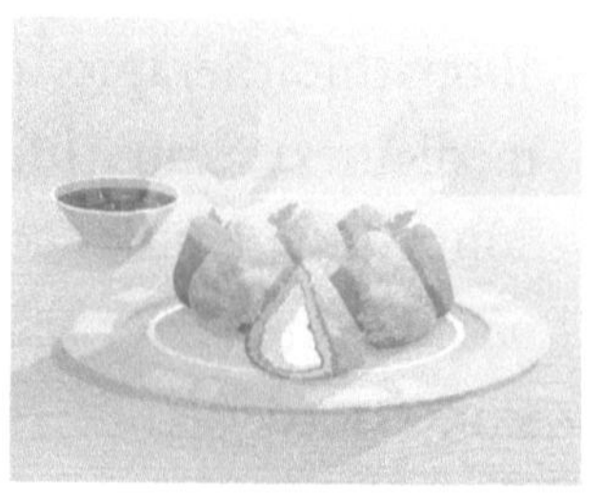

In Ayurveda, diet is very important, and eating things that exacerbate Pitta dosha can lead to acne. Foods that are spicy, fatty, fried, fermented, and acidic can upset the digestive system, causing toxins to build up and skin problems.

Impurities and Toxicity (Ama)

The buildup of toxins and impurities, or "Ama" as it is known in Ayurveda, can obstruct the channels and throw off the equilibrium of the doshas. Poor digestion, erratic eating patterns, or eating unsuitable meal combinations may lead to ama development.

Unbalanced Hormones

Hormonal changes have an impact on the health of the skin, according to Ayurveda. A disruption in the dosha balance can cause acne and pimples, especially during puberty, menstrual cycles, or stressful times.

Digestion problems

The appropriate absorption of nutrients and disposal of waste can be hampered by poor digestion, or "Mandagni" in Ayurvedic terminology. Toxins produced by incomplete digestion can lead to skin conditions like acne.

Emotional and stress factors

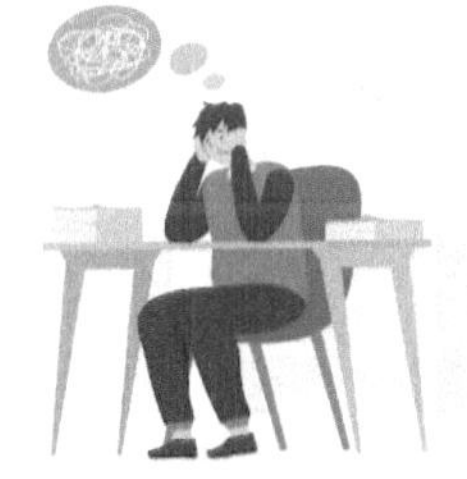

The relationship between the mind and body is emphasized in Ayurveda. The dosha balance can be upset by emotional stress, worry, and an overabundance of mental labor, which can harm skin health and perhaps cause pimples.

Inadequate hygiene

Dirt, extra oil, and dead skin cells can gather on the surface of the skin as a result of improper skincare and cleaning procedures. This may clog the pores and promote the growth of zits.

Seasonal Variations

Seasonal variations' effects on the health of the skin are taken into account by ayurveda. The dosha balance can be upset by changing seasons, especially from winter to spring, and this can result in skin conditions like acne.

Genetic Propensity

According to Ayurveda, a person's Prakriti (constitution) is a key factor in determining how susceptible they are to specific health problems. An individual may be more prone to skin issues like pimples if their prakriti is Pitta-dominant.

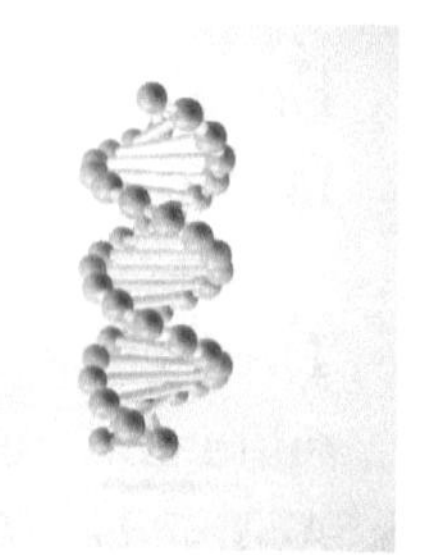

A lot of sun exposure

According to Ayurveda, excessive sun exposure, especially during the height of the day, might worsen Pitta dosha.

This may cause skin irritation and the appearance of pimples.

Changes in Hormones During Puberty

According to Ayurveda, the hormonal surge of puberty, which corresponds to a time of increased Pitta activity, is a typical time for the start of pimples.

Conclusion:

According to Ayurveda, pimples are a reflection of dosha imbalances, especially Pitta, as well as dietary practices, lifestyle decisions, emotional states, and environmental influences. The dosha balance may be restored and pimples can be effectively managed by addressing these underlying causes through a comprehensive approach that includes food change, stress reduction, correct skincare, and adequate cleaning. To attain optimum skin health, Ayurveda promotes an individualized treatment strategy that works with each person's particular constitution and imbalances.

Questions to ask yourself if you have Pimples

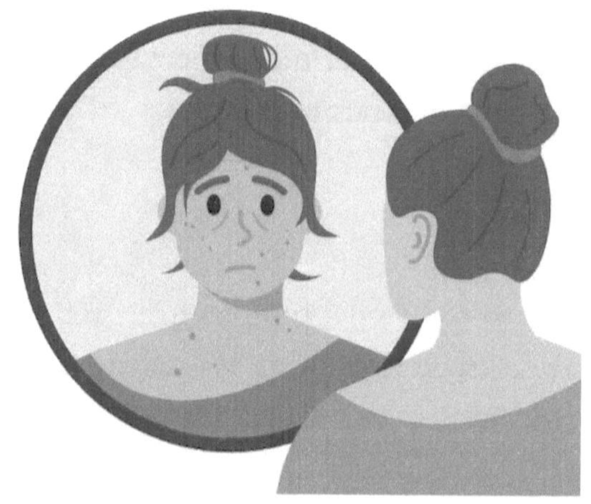

A thorough history-taking procedure is essential in functional and integrative medicine in order to identify the underlying causes of acne and create a personalized treatment strategy. Instead of only treating symptoms, this method focuses on a person's particular biological, psychological, environmental, and behavioral factors to find fundamental causes.

Knowing the patient's medical background:

General Medical History: Start by learning about the patient's general health, prior illnesses, operations, allergies, and prescription drugs. Knowing the patient's medical history might help identify any possible links between past health problems and present skin diseases like acne.

Family Medical History: Find out about your family's medical history, paying specific attention to any skin disorders or acne-related histories. It may be quite helpful to discover probable acne causes by taking into account genetic predispositions and family medical histories.

Evaluation of Lifestyle Factors

Examine the patient's regular eating habits, taking note of if they include processed foods, dairy products, high-glycemic meals, and sugary foods. Hormonal balance and skin health can be substantially impacted by dietary habits.

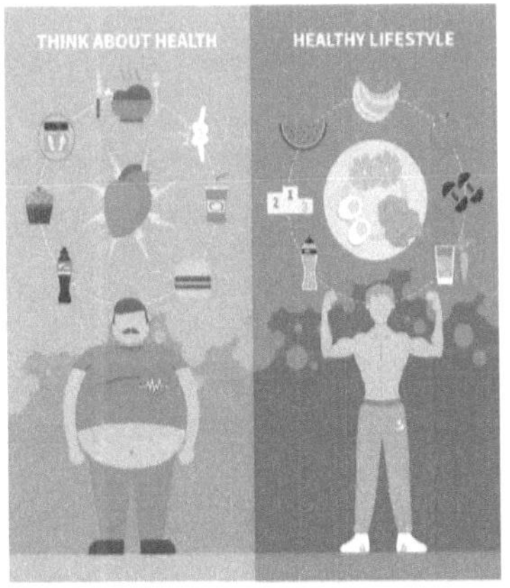

Examine the patient's sleep patterns to find out about their consistency, length, and any abnormalities. For the control of hormones, the reduction of stress, and general skin renewal, a good night's sleep is essential.

Ask the patient about their stress levels, stressors, coping strategies, and lifestyle stressors (such as their workload and personal issues). Hormonal imbalances and acne can both be exacerbated by long-term stress.

Learn about the patient's workout regimen and degree of physical activity. Regular exercise may help with stress management and circulation, both of which are good for skin health.

Menstrual cycle history and hormones:

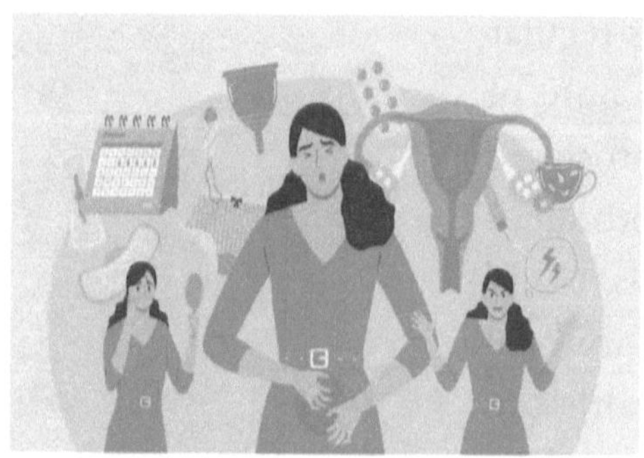

Obtain information on a patient's menstrual cycle, hormonal changes, premenstrual symptoms, and any connections between these factors and acne flare-ups from female patients. The development of acne is frequently significantly influenced by hormonal abnormalities.

If you experience a premenstrual flare of pimples it may be a good idea to discuss with your treating dermatologist to temporarily take oral antihistamines for a few days prior to periods, this in many cases reduces pre menstrual aggravation of acne. Avoid any such practices on your own. Also such approaches may not offer a substitute to root cause approach and treating the real causes, but may be a great option when one is not in a position to make significant lifestyle changes.

Complete Skin Health Evaluation:

Acne History: Gather comprehensive information on the patient's acne, including its development, progression, places on the body, severity, triggers, and any prior therapies. This aids in determining the severity and effects of acne on the patient.

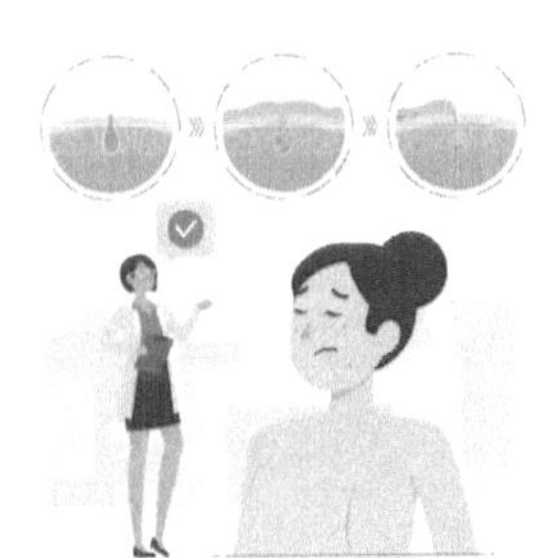

Skin care routine: Examine the patient's existing skincare routine, taking note of the items used, how frequently they are used, and any negative responses. Finding possible irritating variables might be made easier by understanding their skincare routines.

Factors related to the digestive system and diet:

Digestive health: Investigate the patient's digestive health, including bloating, indigestion, and food intolerances. Also look into the patient's bowel motions. A number of skin disorders, including acne, have been related to gut health.

Dietary Sensitivities: Find out if there are any dietary intolerances or allergies that might make acne worse. Certain meals might cause inflammatory reactions and affect the condition of the skin.

Occupational and Environmental Factors:

Exposure to Environmental Toxins: Talk about the patient's everyday exposure to pollutants, chemicals, and environmental toxins. Environmental factors can harm the health of the skin and make acne worse.

Conclusion:

For the purpose of treating acne, a complete history-taking procedure in functional and integrative medicine includes learning about a patient's general health, way of life, hormone patterns, skin health, food, and environmental exposures. Healthcare professionals may create individualized treatment plans that address the underlying causes of acne by taking into account how these factors are interrelated, thus encouraging long-term skin health and general wellbeing.

Beyond only treating the symptoms, this thorough method of identifying and addressing the causes of acne attempts to provide a personalized, holistic strategy for long-term skin health and wellness.

Treatment Options for Pimples in Allopathy

Acne vulgaris, generally known as pimples, is a typical skin disorder that affects a large percentage of people, especially throughout adolescence and the early stages of adulthood. The conventional medical method known as allopathy provides a wide range of effective therapy choices for managing and reducing pimple symptoms. These therapies try to deal with the underlying issues, lessen swelling, manage bacterial development, and avoid scarring. The numerous allopathic treatments for zits are thoroughly examined in this chapter.

Topical remedies:

Benzoyl peroxide: One popular topical acne therapy is benzoyl peroxide. It has anti-inflammatory qualities in addition to working by lowering the amount of P. acnes bacteria on the skin.

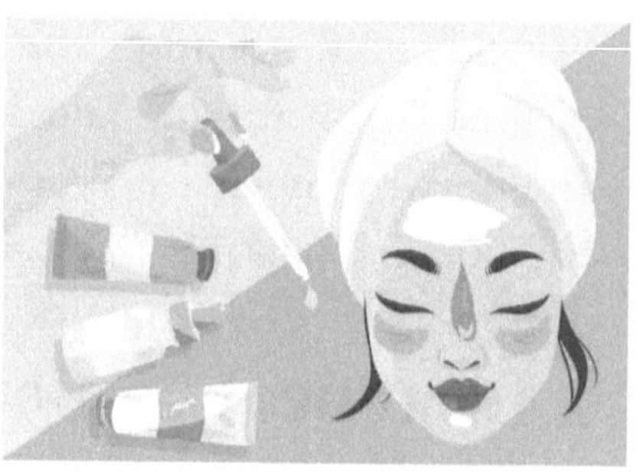

Benzoyl peroxide is sold over-the-counter and comes in different strengths

I PERSONALLY almost always advise patients to do a test patch for benzoyl peroxide before they use it on a larger area. As some of the first time users may be really allergic to it, and if there is an allergy breakout due to this it further affects the patient. So for first time users it is best to use it on a small spot and see in 2-3 days that they are not reacting to it. Allergy to benzoyl peroxide is different from dryness and irritation it can cause. Dryness and slight redness may settle in slowly and are dose and duration dependent, whereas allergies will present more violently and within 1-3 days of first time use and will always be there each time one applies it irrespective of the brand or preparation strength.

You may read further (17)

Topical antibiotics: Topical medications for acne, such as clindamycin, erythromycin, and dapsone, are beneficial.

They function by preventing bacterial development and lowering swelling in the afflicted regions.

It is always best to combine topical antibiotics with benzoyl peroxide so that the acne causing germs do not become resistant. Such practices may help in reducing the overall use of oral antibiotics.

Retinoids: Vitamin A-derived retinoids, such as tretinoin, adapalene, and tazarotene, are effective acne treatments. They assist with pore cleaning, acne prevention, and cell turnover.

*The safest retinoid to apply for acne is **adapalene** and **trifarotene**.*

Topical salicylic acid: Salicylic acid aids in pore cleaning by dissolving oil and dead skin cells. Numerous over-the-counter and prescription topical therapies for pimples utilize it extensively.

Drugs used orally:

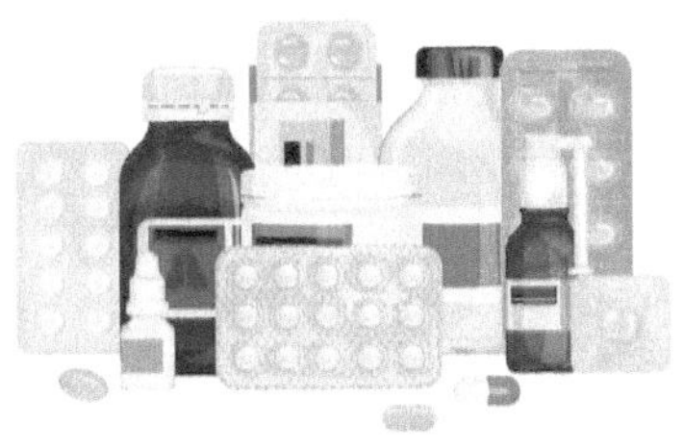

Oral Antibiotics: Patients with moderate to severe acne are given oral antibiotics such tetracycline, doxycycline, and minocycline. They function by lessening inflammation and preventing bacterial growth.

I personally try to minimize the use of oral antibiotics and have found that there is generally not much of a difference in time taken to respond for most patients with or without oral antibiotics. The AAD also recommends " to keep oral antibiotic use to only moderate and severe acne, and to keep the duration to a minimum."

Combination Oral Contraceptives: For females, some combination oral contraceptives that contain both estrogen and progestin can effectively cure acne by managing the hormonal fluctuations that cause it.

Anti-androgens: Spironolactone, a medication, can be used to lower high levels of androgen in both men and women, which is helpful in treating hormonal acne.

Oral anti inflammatory enzymes- This is especially useful when treating red pain and pustular or cystic acne. They really reduce the time to recovery. The basis of use being the fact that in acne there is localized inflammation happening.The presence of C. Acnes bacteria can trigger inflammatory responses.(18)

Isotretinoin:

Strong oral retinoid isotretinoin, which is frequently sold under the trade name Accutane, is used to treat severe, chronic acne that hasn't responded to previous therapies. It treats a number of factors that contribute to acne formation, including excessive oil production, irritation, and P. acnes presence.

Procedures:

Chemical Peels: In a chemical peel, the top layer of skin is removed by applying a chemical solution to the skin. This promotes smoother skin by clearing clogged pores, lowering irritation, and decreasing swelling.

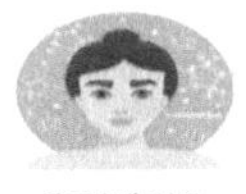
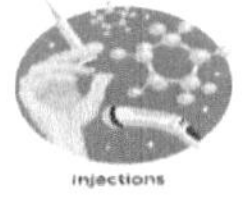
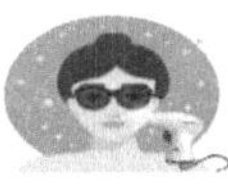

Even though there are a host of new peels for acne and some of them do work very well, one of my evergreen favorites has been the salicylic and mandelic peels which work very well for inflammatory acne. Another peel that works well is the **succinic-azelaic-tranexamic** *combinations by an european brand. While choosing a peel it is important to not to use a very acidic peel ph. As very acidic ph peels may cause a down time and trigger further inflammation in some cases. So what I recommend is the use of lower concentration peels to balance safety and efficacy. Another important TIP to consider before you go in for a peel is that , there should not be any significant dryness, sun burn or irritation on the skin , as that may significantly enhance peel penetration and can be a cause of adverse effects of the peel. So if you have active seborrhoeic dermatitis or are sunburnt just after a vacation it may not be the best time for a peel.*

Microdermabrasion: This procedure employs a machine to mechanically exfoliate the top layer of skin, which helps to clear clogged pores and get rid of dead skin cells. It works well to treat acne that is mild to moderate.

Laser and Light Therapy: A number of laser and light-based therapies, including as photodynamic therapy (PDT), can successfully target the bacteria that cause acne and lessen swelling.

There is some evidence to support for such therapies but the intensity and the number of LEDS used per mask is

important to assess, also it is time taking and has to be used 2-4 times a week at a dose of 5-1.2 j/cm2 dose may work well for 10-30 minutes for best responses, this may reduce compliance.(19)

Additional Therapies:

Comedone Extractor: During an office visit, dermatologists utilize specialized instruments to extract comedones (blackheads and whiteheads), helping to clear the debris from blocked pores.

Intralesional Corticosteroid Injections: To quickly reduce inflammation and enhance healing, corticosteroids can be injected directly into the lesion for big, uncomfortable pimples.

Care and caution must be taken while injecting this. In some cases it can aggravate infection while suppressing the body's inflammatory response. So where needed oral and topical antibiotic cover must be used. Also if overdone it can lead to white/atrophic light coloured scarring. The dose of

triamcinolone used should be minimal to approx 2.5mg/ml and .05-.1 ml per cystic lesion.Never self inject, speak to a doctor experienced in using such procedures.

A wide range of topical and oral drugs, as well as other procedures and complementary therapies, are available as allopathic treatments for pimples. Based on the kind and severity of the acne, the patient's preferences, medical history, and probable side effects, the best course of therapy is chosen. The efficacy and safety of the selected treatment method must be taken into account when developing a customized treatment plan that suits the unique needs of each patient.

In addition to medical therapies, proper skin care practices, a balanced diet, and stress management can enhance the efficacy of allopathic treatments for acne management and skin health in general.

Please be aware that this review only offers a broad grasp of the allopathic treatment choices for zits and should not be used as a substitute for consulting a doctor. For individualized advice and care, always seek the advice of a healthcare expert.

Integrative Medical Approach to Treating Acne

Acne, a widespread dermatological disorder that affects millions of people worldwide, has traditionally been treated using a variety of medical methods. A distinct viewpoint on comprehending and treating acne is provided by the holistic and patient-centered Integrative Medical Approach. Integrative medicine examines the interactions between several factors, including nutrition, lifestyle, gut health, hormonal balance, and stress, in an effort to pinpoint the underlying causes of illnesses, including acne. In-depth discussion of the Integrative Medical Approach's method for treating acne by addressing underlying imbalances and fostering general wellbeing is provided in this chapter.

Gut health and Acne

Gut microbiome: According to research, there is a direct link between acne and the gut microbiota. An imbalance in intestinal bacteria known as dysbiosis can cause inflammation and skin problems. The 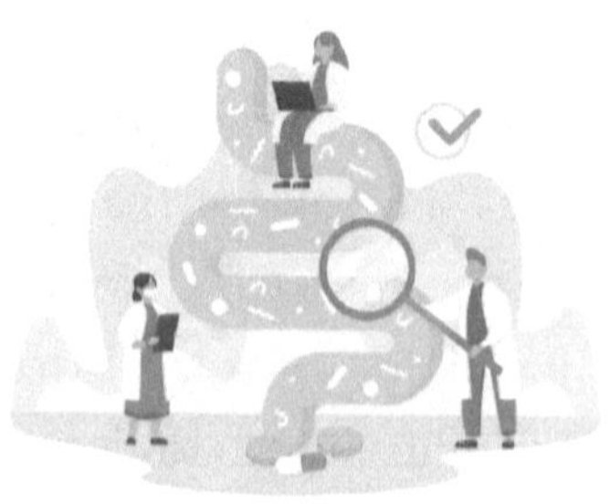 Integrative Medical Approach places a strong emphasis on improving gut health through a balanced diet, probiotics, and treating digestive problems.

There are certain types of gut microbiomes described which can impact the inflammatory or anti inflammatory mediators circulating in our bodies.

Leaky Gut Syndrome: A "leaky gut" permits bacteria and poisons to enter the circulation, setting off an inflammatory reaction that may take the form of acne. Through dietary adjustments and gut-healing regimens, the Integrative Medical Approach treats leaky gut to lessen inflammation and enhance skin health.

Acne and hormonal balance

Insulin Resistance: Elevated insulin levels and insulin resistance can promote acne-causing inflammation and excessive sebum production. To increase insulin sensitivity and control acne, the Integrative Medical Approach focuses on food changes, exercise, and blood sugar regulation.([20](#), [21](#),[22](#), [23](#), [24](#))

Addition of specific types of fasting methods significantly helps in reducing acne outbreaks and rapidly reduces inflammation. Fasting may be of one meal a day , or intermittent or complete 24 hr water fast. It is best to proceed with the fasts under supervision only. Addition of some herbs, spices like cinnamon and medicines like metformin for a short course always help in insulin sensitivity.

Balance between estrogen and testosterone: Hormonal disorders, particularly those caused by excessive amounts of androgens like testosterone, can make acne worse. The Integrative Medical Approach uses nutritional therapies, stress management techniques, and lifestyle changes to help regulate hormones.

Inflammation and acne

Dietary Inflammatory Triggers: Some meals, particularly those heavy in unhealthy fats and processed carbohydrates, can cause inflammation and exacerbate acne. An anti-inflammatory diet high in fruits, vegetables, omega-3 fatty acids, and antioxidants is recommended by the Integrative Medical Approach.

Inflammation and Stress: Prolonged stress can exacerbate inflammation, which exacerbates acne. The Integrative Medical Approach uses methods for reducing stress including yoga, meditation, and mindfulness to control inflammation and enhance skin health.

Just focusing on sleep hygiene and improving sleep quality and quantity with herbs like centella asiatica etc goes a long way in some patients to reduce their stress levels.

Acne detoxification

Toxic Load: According to the Integrative Medical Approach, a healthy body must be able to get rid of toxins. Acne management requires optimal liver function and the assistance of detoxification pathways.

Environmental Toxins: Being exposed to environmental toxins might throw off your hormones and make you break out in acne. The Integrative Medical Approach places a strong emphasis on minimizing exposure to toxins and assisting the body's own detoxification processes.

Personalized dietary strategies

The Integrative Medical Approach takes individualized treatments based on a person's particular biochemistry, allergies, sensitivities, and gut health and acknowledges the effect of nutrition on acne. Common dietary changes could involve staying away from dairy, gluten, and processed foods.

Dietary exclusion is very different for different patients and needs a comprehensive understanding as per body type. For example for a vata dominant person with severe acne, it may be detrimental to completely stop dairy and non vegetarian foods. Whereas in a pitta person it may be more important to stop intake of chili and coffee, tea etc type of stimulant foods. This is the same reason why in western medicine we often see conflicting information about the role of diet in different studies. If we learn a bit more about the ayurvedic body type concept we can more accurately predict and understand what works and what doesn't for our body.

Stress management- role of psychological stress in aggravating hormone imbalance is well established. A customized plan to bring attention to stress management may help. The role of stress is well established.

Here is something interesting to read: *The response of skin disease to stress: changes in the severity of acne vulgaris as affected by examination stress.* ([25](#))([26](#))

Conclusion:

By addressing the underlying causes of acne rather than just treating the symptoms, the holistic Medical Approach provides a thorough and holistic approach to treating the condition. The Integrative Medical Approach aims to maximize overall health, successfully treating and preventing acne by concentrating on gut health, hormonal balance, inflammation reduction, detoxification, and tailored dietary programs.

A healthcare provider with expertise in the Integrative Medical Approach should be consulted in order to create a customized treatment plan that takes into account each patient's particular requirements and circumstances.

This review does not replace seeking expert medical advice; rather, it gives a broad knowledge of the Integrative Medical Approach to managing acne. For individualized advice and care, always seek the advice of a healthcare expert.

CHAPTER 10:
HAIRFALL

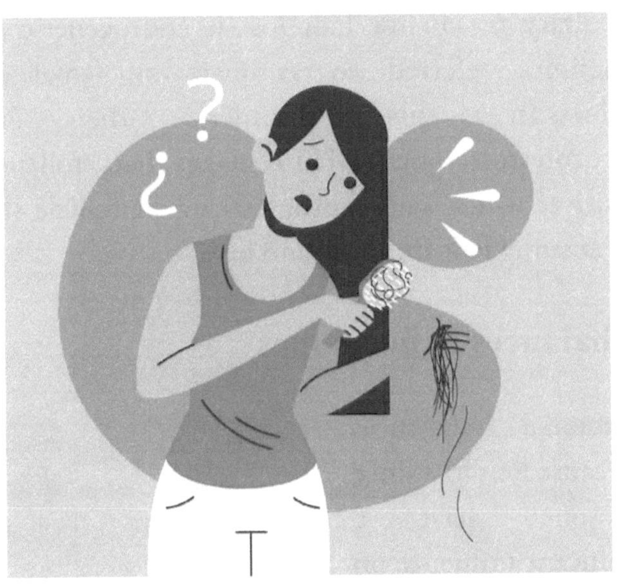

Hair Loss Causes According to Allopathy

Alopecia, or hair loss, is a prevalent problem that impacts people of all ages and genders. The modern medical theory of health known as allopathy provides a thorough grasp of the numerous variables causing hair loss. This chapter explores the main reasons for hair loss according to allopathic medicine, illuminating the science and medical viewpoint behind this common problem.

Genetic Elements

An individual's propensity for hair loss is significantly influenced by hereditary factors. The most prevalent hereditary reason for hair loss is androgenetic alopecia, sometimes referred to as male or female pattern baldness.In this disorder, the hormone dihydrotestosterone (DHT) makes hair follicles more sensitive, which causes progressive hair follicle shrinkage and ensuing hair thinning and loss.

Imbalances in hormones

Hormonal imbalances can cause hair loss since hormones have a significant influence on hair health. Key hormonal elements linked to hair loss include:

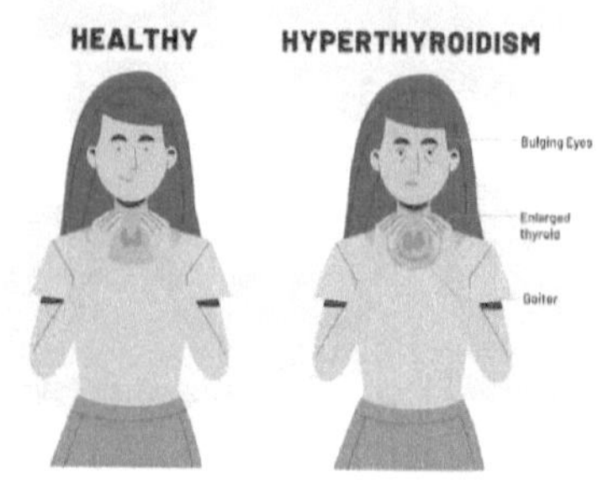

Disorders of the thyroid: Hair loss can result from thyroid conditions such as hypothyroidism (an underactive thyroid) and hyperthyroidism (an overactive thyroid).

Polycystic Ovary Syndrome (PCOS): PCOS is a common hormonal condition in women that frequently causes significant hair loss because of increased androgen levels.

Menopause: Women who are going through menopause may have hair loss and thinning due to hormonal changes.

Nutritional Insufficiencies

Essential nutrients can make hair brittle and cause hair loss. The following are typical dietary deficits that cause hair loss.

Iron Deficiency: Hair thinning and severe hair loss can be caused by anemia brought on by a low iron consumption.

Vitamin D Deficiency: Low vitamin D levels have been linked to hair loss and may have an impact on the health of hair follicles.

Protein Deficiency: Because keratin, a kind of protein, makes up the majority of hair, a diet low in protein can make hair brittle and increase hair loss.

Medications and Medical Conditions

Hair loss is a side effect of a number of illnesses and drugs. Typical illustrations include:

Autoimmune diseases: When an autoimmune disorder like lupus or alopecia areata is present, the immune system may wrongly attack hair follicles, resulting in hair loss.

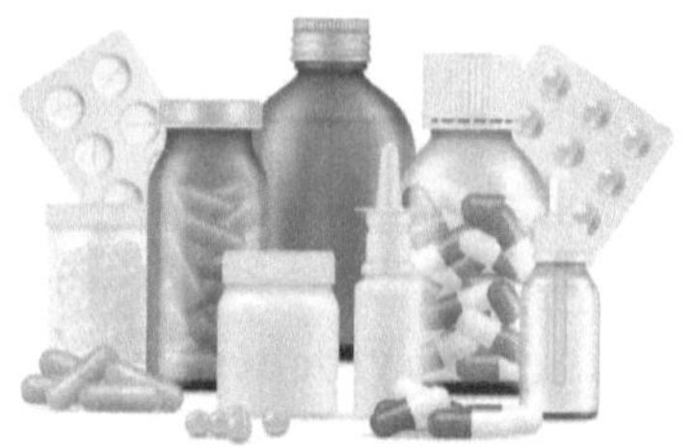

Chemotherapy and radiation treatment are essential for treating cancer, but they also frequently cause hair loss because they damage rapidly dividing cells, such as hair follicles.

Drugs: Hair loss is a potential adverse effect of certain medications, including those for high blood pressure, depression, and birth control.

Stress, both physical and emotional

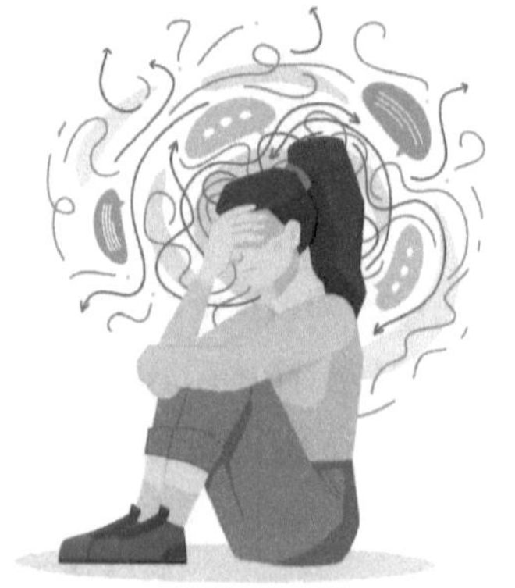

Telogen effluvium is a disorder that results from the disruption of the hair growth cycle by physical and mental stress. A higher proportion of hair follicles than typical enter the resting phase at this stage and eventually fall out. Hair loss brought on by stress is frequently just temporary, and after the underlying stressor is resolved, hair growth usually returns.

Poor Hair Care Practices:

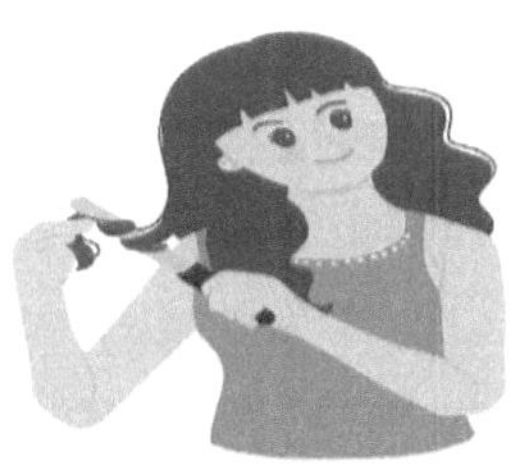

Hair damage and hair loss can be caused by excessive style, heat styling, chemical treatments, and regular usage of hair products. The necessity of gentle hair care techniques to reduce the risk of hair loss is emphasized by allopathy.

According to allopathic medicine, there are many different factors that might contribute to hair loss, including genetics, hormonal imbalances, nutritional deficiencies, illnesses, drugs, stress, and incorrect hair care techniques. For effective treatment strategies to be developed, it is essential to understand the underlying causes of hair loss. Consult a dermatologist or healthcare provider as soon as you notice hair loss so they can do a comprehensive assessment and suggest the best course of action for your unique situation.

Hair Loss Factors According to Ayurveda

The traditional Indian medical system of Ayurveda provides a comprehensive explanation of the reasons for hair loss. According to Ayurveda, imbalances in the doshas—the underlying forces that guide our bodies—have an impact on hair health, which is strongly linked to one's whole state of health. Ayurveda has several theories on why people lose their hair, taking into account both internal and external influences. This chapter explores the many causes of hair loss from an Ayurvedic perspective.

Unbalanced Dosha:

Vata, Pitta, and Kapha are the three doshas according to Ayurveda. Asymmetry in certain doshas is frequently linked to hair loss:

1. Vata Imbalance: The exacerbated Vata dosha can cause dryness, poor blood flow, and weak hair follicles. As a result, hair may become dry, brittle, and more fragile.

Hair loss and receding hair line is attributable to vata imbalance, sometimes accompanied by dryness of scalp and dry skin, family history of heart diseases and or diabetic tendency in the individual or first family.

2. Pitta Imbalance: Too much Pitta dosha can cause a rise in body temperature, which may harm the hair follicles. Due to the high temperatures and inflammation, it may cause premature graying, hair thinning, and hair loss.

Early graying and hair thinning is generally attributed to pitta imbalances.

3. Kapha Imbalance: Imbalance in the Kapha dosha can cause the scalp to become too oily and congested, thereby obstructing hair follicles and causing hair loss.

Poor nutrition and diet:

Ayurveda places a strong emphasis on the value of a nutritious and well-balanced diet for good hair. Hair loss may be brought on by:

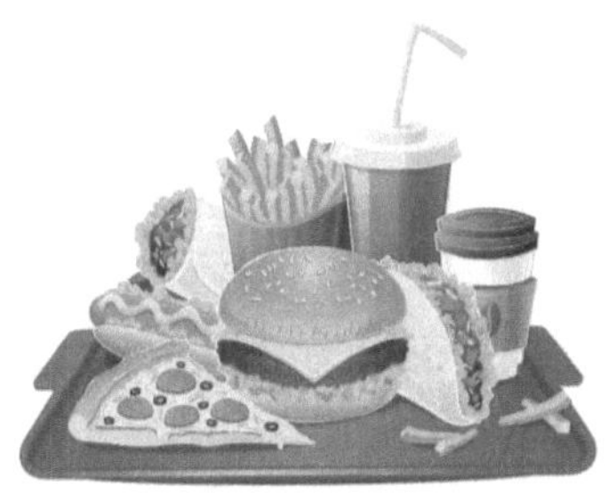

- **Poor Nutrition:** Weak hair and hair loss can result from a diet lacking in vital elements such proteins, vitamins, and minerals.
- **Foods that are too hot and salty:** Eating too many spicy and salty foods might irritate Pitta dosha, which may cause hair loss.

- **Food Allergies:** Undiagnosed dietary sensitivities or allergies can cause inflammation and hair loss.

Even in modern medicine, the role of nutrition and nutritional supplementation is well established. The role of zinc, iron, ferritin and many other micronutrients is well established.

Emotional and stress-related factors:

The relationship between the mind and body is acknowledged in ayurveda. The dosha equilibrium can be upset by stress, worry, and emotional instability, which can cause hair loss:

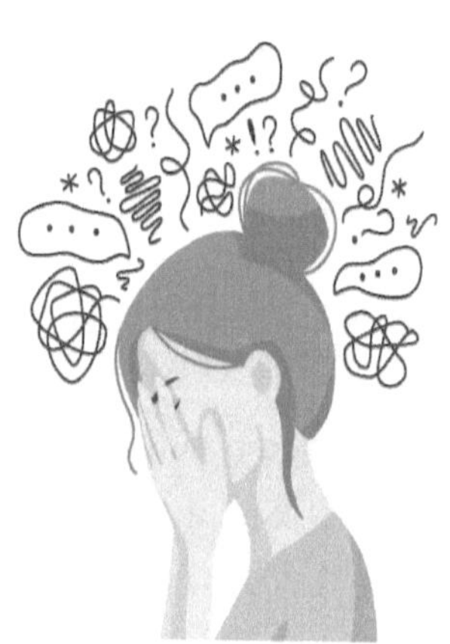

- **Long-term stress:** Pitta dosha can be aggravated by chronic stress, which might result in hair loss.

- **Emotional Imbalances:** Dosha imbalances caused by unresolved emotional difficulties can have an impact on the health of one's hair.

Unwise lifestyle choices:

- **Lack of Sleep:** Lack of sleep can interfere with the body's normal healing processes and dosha balance, which can affect the health of the hair.

Chronic lack of sleep is a potent stressor on the body and not only does it disturb the steroid secretion and circadian rhythms but it also impacts insulin related metabolism and in many patients also leads to frequent digestive symptoms. Chronic sleep deprivation may interfere with absorption of food in the gastrointestinal system too. For some of our patients when the sleep cycle is corrected for a period of only 2-4 weeks they begin noting a significant improvement in their digestive symptoms which inturn will also lead to assisting in skin and hair quality.

- **Excessive exercise:** Excessive exercise, particularly when it results in excessive perspiration, might upset Pitta dosha and cause hair loss.

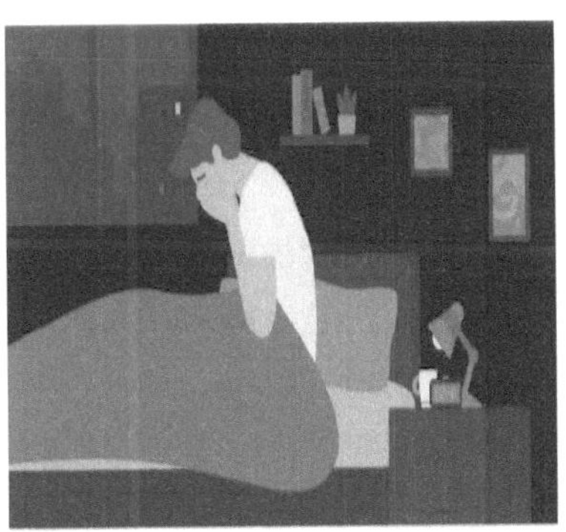

- **Unreliable Routine:** Unreliable daily routines can impact hair loss and disrupt the equilibrium of the body as a whole.

Scalp Wellness:

- **Insufficient Scalp Hygiene:** Dirt, extra oil, and dandruff can build up on the scalp due to improper cleaning and upkeep, which is bad for the health of the hair.
- **Chemical-laden hair products:** Using harsh or chemical-rich hair products can harm the hair and scalp, which can lead to hair loss.

This is much understated, poorly understood and often neglected in evaluations. As a single hair care product contains a number of ingredients , on an average 2-3 hair care products are used, the exposure from such products can have significant impacts on the hair shaft and scalp.

Environmental elements

- **Excessive sun exposure:** Overexposure to the sun can exacerbate Pitta dosha and cause hair issues, especially if it occurs during peak hours.

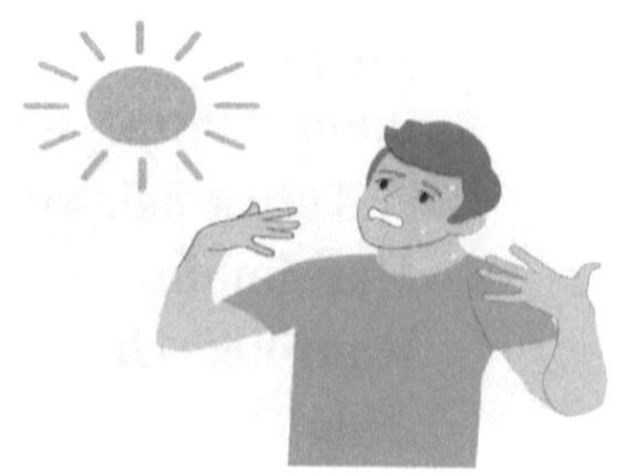

To tackle this concern in modern medicine, only recently have we been talking about and recommending hair sunscreens, but the long term effects and efficacy of such products is still far from established.

- **Environmental Toxins:** The dosha balance can be upset and the hair gets negatively impacted by exposure to pollution, chemicals, and toxins.

Imbalance of hormones

The equilibrium of the doshas can be upset by hormonal fluctuations, such as those that occur during pregnancy, menopause, or medical illnesses like polycystic ovarian syndrome (PCOS), which can result in hair loss.

Genetic Propensity:

According to Ayurveda, a person's Prakriti (constitution) might affect how susceptible they are to hair loss. A Pitta-dominant Prakriti may be more prone to premature

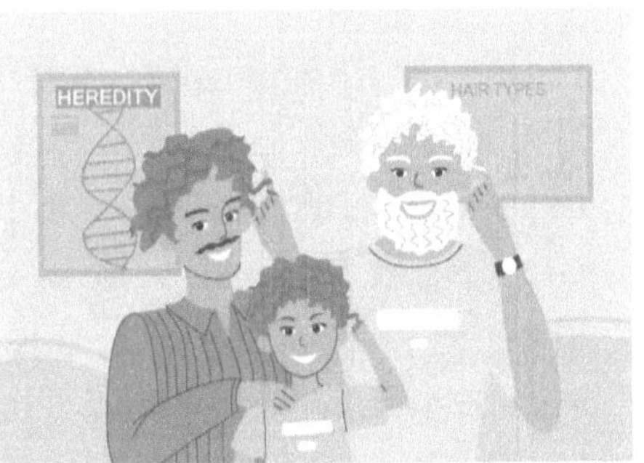

graying and hair loss, whereas a Vata-dominant Prakriti may be more prone to dry, brittle hair.

According to Ayurveda, hair loss is a sign of dosha imbalances, which are impacted by a person's nutrition, way of life, emotional state, environment, and genetic predispositions. Ayurveda promotes a customized therapy strategy that is in line with a person's particular constitution and imbalances in order to address the underlying reasons of hair loss. This strategy entails nutritional changes, stress reduction, appropriate hair care, and lifestyle alterations. Ayurveda offers a complete plan for preventing and managing hair fall, encouraging healthy and glossy hair by reestablishing dosha equilibrium and fostering general wellbeing.

Questions to ask yourself if you have hair fall problem

People of all ages and genders are concerned about hair loss, which is a common problem. It's important to start by asking yourself a series of questions that might provide you insight into the various reasons for your hair fall in order to successfully treat this issue. These inquiries cover a wide variety of topics, including your lifestyle, general health, and environmental exposures. You can identify the underlying causes of hair loss by pondering on these questions and working to find the best management and prevention strategies.

Questions on general health and lifestyle:

1. Have You Been Eating Balanced? Examine the quality of your food and if it offers your body the proteins, vitamins, and minerals it needs to support the growth of healthy hair.

2. Are You Under Stress? Consider your level of stress and how it may be affecting your entire health, including the condition of your hair.

3. Are You Getting Enough Sleep? Examine your sleeping habits and ask yourself if you're giving your body enough time to recover so that it can continue to produce healthy hair.

4. Is your routine dependable? Consider how consistent your daily routine is. Consistencies may damage the health of your hair by upsetting the equilibrium of your body as a whole.

5. How active Are You? Think about your degree of exercise. Finding the appropriate balance is essential since both excessive and insufficient physical activity can have an impact on hair health.

Questions about hair care and styling

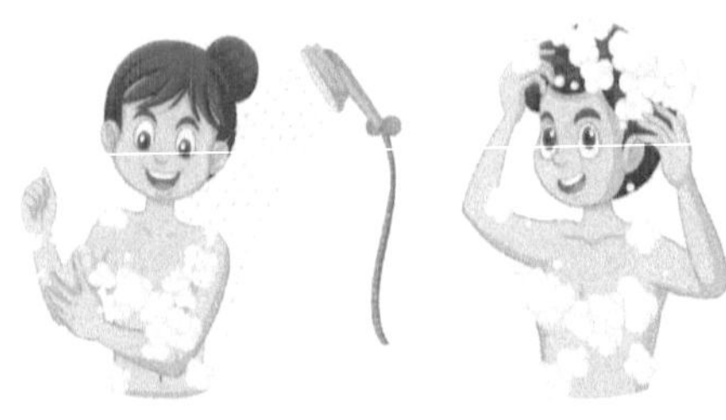

1. How Do You Take Care of Your Hair? Analyze the hair products you use often, paying close attention to shampoos, conditioners, and style aids. Verify your environment for any harsh chemicals or irritants that can be causing hair loss.

2. What Is Your Hair Washing Routine? Assess how often you wash your hair. Your hair's health can be negatively impacted by both over- and under-washing.

3. Are You Overheating Your Hair? Consider how often you use hot styling equipment like curling irons, straighteners, or hair dryers. An excessive amount of heat styling can harm hair and cause hair fall.

4. Are You Tying Your Hair Tightly? Consider your options for hairstyles, such as braids or tight ponytails. These may cause the hair to get strained and break.

5. Do You Color Your Hair or Treat It? Think about how regularly you color, perm, or otherwise treat your hair chemically. Over time, these processes may cause the hair to deteriorate.

Scalp Hygiene and Health Issues

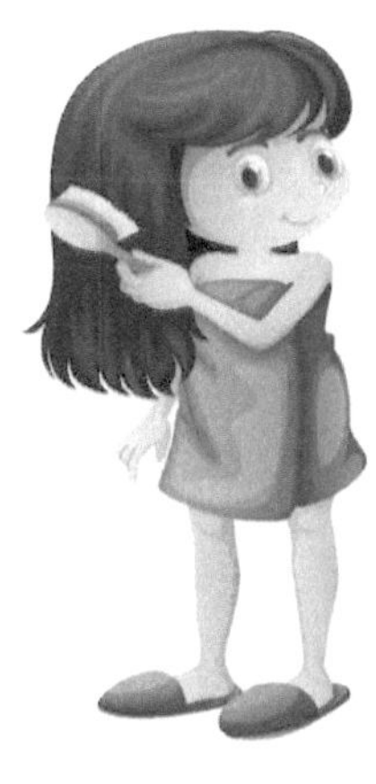

1. Do You Have a Clean, Healthy Scalp? Check your scalp for any indications of problems like dandruff, itchiness, or excessive oiliness because these disorders can cause hair loss.

2. How frequently do you comb or brush your hair? Review your hair-care routine, paying particular attention to how you treat your hair. Hair can break when brushed or combed harshly.

3. Have You Noticed Any Changes in the Texture of Your Hair? Pay attention to any changes in your hair that may be precursors to hair loss, such as thinning, dryness, or brittleness.

4. Are You Receiving Medical Care? It's crucial to understand that medical treatments, such as chemotherapy, might affect the health of your hair if you're presently undergoing them.

5. Do you often get painful or itchy eruptions on the scalp?

Genetics and Family:

Is Hair Loss in the Family a Problem? Look into if hair thinning or loss runs in your family. Your predisposition to hair loss may be significantly influenced by your genetics.

Medical and Hormonal Issues:

1. Has Your Hormone Level Recently Changed? Consider any recent hormonal changes that may have caused hair loss, such as those brought on by menopause, pregnancy, or other medical disorders.

2. Do You Suffer From Any Medical Conditions? Consider whether you have any underlying health issues that could be impacting your hair, and seek medical advice if necessary.

Environmental elements:

Are Environmental Toxins a Concern for You? Consider your regular exposure to chemicals and pollutants because they can affect the health of your hair and cause hair loss.

Nutrition and Diet:

1. Are You Eating Balancedly? Make sure your meals contain a range of nutrients by evaluating your dietary choices. Lack of nutrition may be a factor in hair loss.

Eating processed food is a big challenge, do observe how much of packaged and processed food you consume versus fresh cooked and whole foods.

2. Do You Have Food Sensitivities or Allergies? Take into account whether you have any underlying dietary sensitivities or allergies that might be resulting in follicle inflammation and hair loss. It could be important to seek advice from an allergist or medical specialist.

You'll learn a lot about the possible reasons for your hair loss as you reflect on these questions. In order to treat and manage hair loss, it is important to first identify the underlying causes.

While these self-reflection questions are a good place to start, it's crucial to speak with a dermatologist or healthcare provider for a full assessment and advice that are specialized for your unique circumstances.

Treatment options for hair loss in allopathy

People of all ages and genders worry about hair loss, which may be upsetting and influence one's self-esteem. The traditional medical approach known as allopathy provides a number of therapy options to address the root causes of hair loss and encourage hair regeneration. We shall examine the thorough allopathic management alternatives for treating hair fall in this chapter.

1. Drugs used topically:

a. Minoxidil

One of the most popular topical treatments for hair loss is minoxidil. Both over-the-counter and prescription-strength versions are offered. By boosting blood flow to the hair follicles and lengthening the hair's development phase, minoxidil encourages hair regeneration. Usually applied directly to the scalp, it requires regular, sustained application to maintain benefits.

b. The drug finasteride

An FDA-approved prescription drug for hair loss, especially in males, is finasteride. Dihydrotestosterone (DHT), a hormone known to lead to hair loss, is inhibited in order for it to operate. Finasteride promotes regrowth and slows hair loss, but it has possible negative effects and should only be used under medical supervision.

2. Drugs used orally:

a. Finasteride (brand name Propecia):

As previously indicated, the main target population for the prescription oral drug finasteride is males suffering from androgenetic alopecia. It aids in lessening DHT's negative effects on hair follicles, decreasing hair loss and promoting regeneration.

b. Spironolactone:

Another oral medicine used off-label for females with androgenetic alopecia is spironolactone. It functions by lessening androgens' (male hormones) impact on hair follicles.

c. Anti-androgens:

Anti-androgen drugs may occasionally be prescribed by medical practitioners to reduce hair loss by lessening the impact of hormones like DHT on the hair follicles. These drugs could include flutamide and cyproterone acetate.

3. Stimulants for hair growth:

a. LLLT, or low-level laser therapy:

By stimulating hair follicles with red light producing devices or laser caps, low-level laser therapy may increase hair density and promote hair growth. LLLT can be used in a clinical environment or at home.

b. Therapy with platelet-rich plasma (PRP):

A tiny amount of the patient's blood is drawn, processed to obtain platelet-rich plasma, and then injected into the scalp as part of PRP treatment. Growth factors included in PRP have the ability to stimulate hair follicles, increase hair thickness, and promote regeneration.

4. Hair Replacement:

a. FUT (Follicular Unit Transplantation):

FUT, sometimes referred to as strip surgery, entails the removal of a strip of scalp from the donor area, its subsequent dissection into individual follicular units, and its subsequent transplantation into the recipient area. For

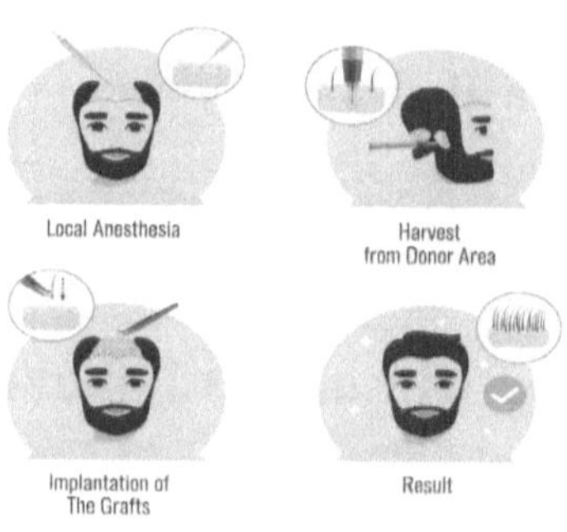

concealing greater regions of hair loss, use this technique.

b. FUE, or Follicular Unit Extraction:

Individual hair follicles are removed from the donor region and transplanted to the recipient area using the minimally invasive hair transplantation procedure known as FUE. Compared to FUT, it produces less scars and has a speedier recovery.

5. Scalp Sizing

In a surgical operation called a "scalp reduction," a portion of the bald scalp is removed, and the skin next to it is stretched to cover the region. Large bald patches are addressed with this technique.

Since the advent and advances in hair transplant techniques , this is seldom used for regular types of hair loss. Only in some types of hair loss like scarring, or post traumatic this may be advocated.

6. Complementary Therapies:

a. Dietary Supplements:

To promote the health of the hair, supplements comprising biotin, vitamins, minerals, and amino acids are frequently advised. Biotin is well known for its contribution to hair growth.

The new concept in dietary supplementation is the use of rotational hair supplements, which is the practice of

adding different supplements in higher doses on different days of the week. This practice mimics our natural nutritional cycles and may help in better absorption of the supplied nutrients.

b. Hair Care Items:

Hair health and hair loss reduction are promoted by shampoos, conditioners, and topical treatments that contain substances like saw palmetto, caffeine, or ketoconazole.

7. Changes to Your Lifestyle:

In order to control hair loss, a healthy lifestyle must be maintained. This involves maintaining a healthy weight, controlling stress, exercising often, and getting enough sleep. These way of life changes can support other therapeutic approaches.

Conclusion:

For controlling hair loss, allopathy provides a variety of treatments, ranging from topical and oral drugs to cutting-edge procedures including hair transplantation and low-level laser therapy. The choice of therapy is influenced by the underlying cause of hair loss, personal considerations, and medical expert advice. To choose the best course of therapy and take care of your unique needs, you must visit a dermatologist or hair expert. Allopathic medicines have a chance to be helpful, but for the greatest outcomes and to reduce potential adverse effects, they should be administered under the guidance of a medical practitioner.

One is often told that if you want to continue to have lush hair, the medication needs to be applied for as long as you want good hair growth, This idea seems flawed, as if we have achieved true homoeostasis and metabolic balance, the regrown hair should stay or at least the reduction in hair fall and pace of hair loss should be maintained in the reduced state.

Integrative Medical Approach to Treating Hair Fall in Men and Women

Men and women both worry about hair loss, which may be upsetting and affect self-esteem. The Integrative Medical Approach, a patient-centered and holistic paradigm, provides a thorough approach to comprehend and treat hair loss by treating the underlying reasons and enhancing general wellbeing. In-depth discussion of the Integrative Medical Approach's comprehensive and multidimensional approach to controlling hair loss is provided in this chapter.

From the perspective of integrative medicine, understanding hair loss:

The Integrative Medical Approach views hair loss as a manifestation of interior bodily imbalances rather than as a separate problem. Hair health is viewed as a reflection of one's general health and the smooth operation of several systems, including the immunological, gastrointestinal, endocrine, and detoxification systems.

Hair loss and gut health:

a. Gut Microbiome:

The gut microbiota and the condition of one's hair are strongly related, according to research. Inflammation and oxidative stress brought on by a gut dysbiosis may result in hair loss. The Integrative Medical Approach places a strong emphasis on eating a balanced diet and taking probiotics and prebiotics to maintain a healthy gut.

It is also a well known fact that if the microbiome is healthy it will assist in better digestion of dietary components and better bioavailability. If there is dysbiosis, the assimilation of nutrients may be impacted which will ultimately impact all tissues, with hair responding faster than many other tissues of the body.

b. Leaky Gut Syndrome

Toxins and bacteria can enter the circulation as a result of leaky gut, a disease in which the intestinal lining becomes porous. An inflammatory reaction may result from this and cause hair loss. Leaky gut is addressed by the Integrative Medical Approach through dietary modifications and gut-healing procedures.

This may more directly to autoimmune type of hair loss, more so than the commonly seen Male and Female pattern hair losses. Leaky gut is being increasingly linked to autoimmunity, which is associated with hair loss labeled as Alopecia areata and telogen effluvium

2. Hormonal equilibrium and hair loss:

a. Hormonal Changes:

Hair loss can be made worse by hormonal imbalances, especially when there are high amounts of androgens like testosterone. The Integrative Medical Approach uses nutritional therapies, stress management techniques, and lifestyle changes to help regulate hormones.

IT IS IMPORTANT TO NOTE THAT- the hormone health is related to the type of food and how it's metabolized by the individual, the role of dairy, gluten, chocolates and sugary foods in

various hormonally driven skin concerns like acne and hair loss are increasingly being established. The hormone health is influenced by
- *food- type of food, quantity, timing of food and food combinations*
- *gut health- the enterotype (microbiome type)*
- *muscle mass and activity levels*
- *tissue oxygenation, breathing and movement levels*
- *deep rest sleep and mental emotional stress, this being one of the most often missed and understated root causes. Here is an interesting read about the concept of microbiome and hormone health.(27)*

b. Thyroid Condition:

Hair health can be impacted by thyroid conditions, including hyperthyroidism and hypothyroidism. To manage hair loss successfully, integrative medicine takes thyroid function into account and works to optimize it.

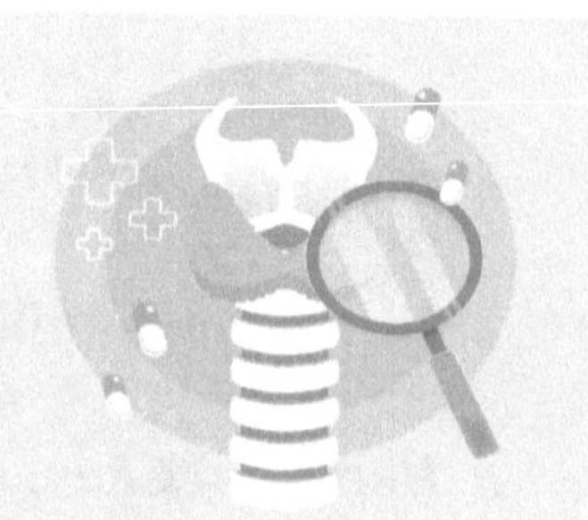

Many patients come with thyroid profiles done, or are on medication, whereas the thyroid profile is normal in most patients as they are on hormone supplementation, but it is not uncommon to find low grade or many times frank anti thyroid antibodies in patients who complain of hair loss.

3. Hair loss and inflammation

a. Foods that cause inflammation:

Certain diets, particularly those heavy in unhealthy fats and refined carbohydrates, can cause inflammation and exacerbate hair loss. An anti-inflammatory diet high in fruits, vegetables, omega-3 fatty acids, and antioxidants is recommended by the Integrative Medical Approach.

The frequent intake of fried snacks, alcohol, processed dairy and processed and packaged food also contributes to inflammation. The role of sugar in triggering inflammation is often understated.

b. Stress and inflammation

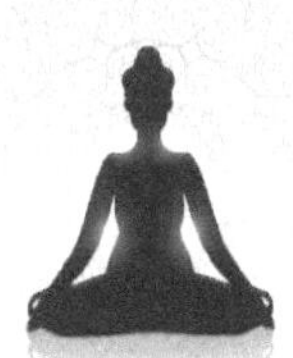

Chronic stress can make inflammation worse, which can cause hair loss. The Integrative Medical Approach uses methods of stress reduction including yoga, meditation, and mindfulness to control inflammation and enhance hair health.

The exact mechanisms of stress, especially emotional stress induced hair loss, are poorly understood, but commonly observed.

4. Detoxification and hair loss

a. The toxic load :

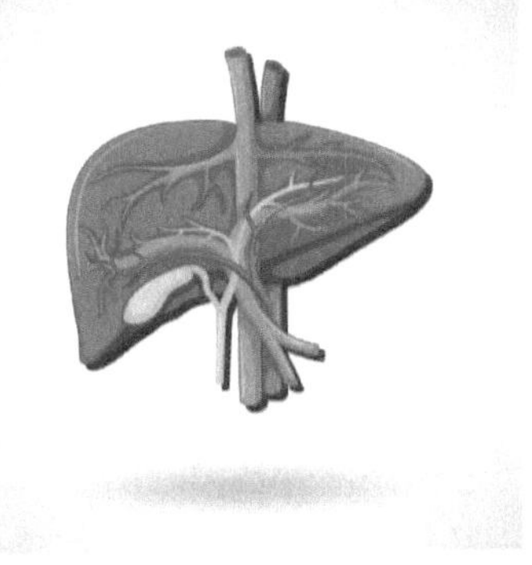

The Integrative Medical Approach acknowledges that keeping healthy hair depends on the body's capacity to get rid of pollutants. In order to control hair loss, detoxification via healthy liver function and supported detox pathways is crucial.

b. Toxins in the environment:

Environmental contaminants can throw off hormonal balance and cause hair loss. The Integrative Medical Approach places a strong emphasis on minimizing exposure to toxins and assisting the body's own detoxification processes.

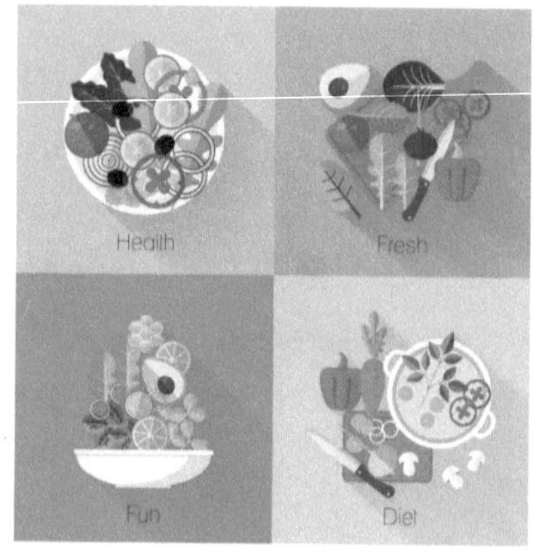

5. Customized dietary strategies:

A tailored food plan based on a person's distinct biochemistry, allergies, sensitivities, and gut health is adopted by the Integrative Medical Approach, which recognizes the influence of nutrition on hair health. Avoiding trigger foods, treating deficiencies, and putting an emphasis on nutrient-dense meals are examples of common dietary adjustments.

6. Dietary supplements:

To promote the health of the hair, supplements comprising biotin, vitamins, minerals, and amino acids are frequently advised. These supplements can be customized to meet each person's unique needs.

Conclusion:

The Integrative Medical Approach focuses on gut health, hormonal balance, inflammation reduction, detoxification, and specific nutritional regimens to address hair loss in a holistic and one-on-one manner. Healthcare professionals may create individualized treatment plans that address the underlying causes of hair loss, advance general wellbeing, and successfully manage and prevent hair loss by taking into account how these factors are interrelated.

To create a tailored treatment plan that takes into account each patient's particular requirements and circumstances, it is crucial to speak with a healthcare expert with expertise in the Integrative Medical Approach. This chapter provides an overview of the Integrative Medical Approach to managing hair loss, but it should not be used as a substitute for seeking competent medical advice. A healthcare expert should always be consulted for specific advice and treatment.

The tailored treatment plan includes
- assessment of the body type
- factors in individual food choices and sensitivities,
- focuses on connecting the patient with their own bodies for a better understanding of the high impact factors causing hair loss
- managing all factors surrounding hair loss like , correcting underlying digestive concerns, aiding better digestion and absorption.
- cutting out inflammatory foods and foods that may hinder absorption of nutrients like tea or coffee along with food.
- assisting in stem cell rejuvenation by using principles of fasting as per ayurveda or chinese medicine body type. For example a vata body type may do a completely different fast or may not be recommended fasting at all whereas a kapha body type may be able to do a more aggressive fast after proper preparation.
- making use of the best of modern dermatological preparations is included for a faster and more comprehensive respect

CHAPTER 11-
FUNGAL SKIN INFECTIONS
AND DANDRUFF

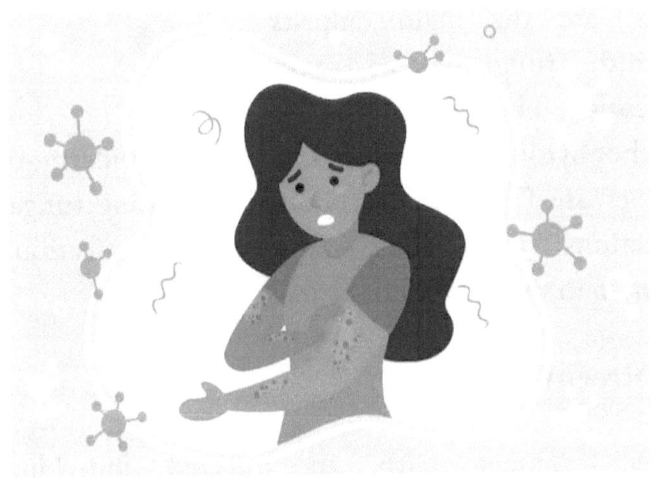

Causes of fungal skin infection according to allopathy-

Dermatophytosis and tinea are other names for fungal skin infections, which are frequent dermatological disorders brought on by different fungi. The standard medical approach known as allopathic medicine acknowledges a number of variables that contribute to the emergence of fungal skin diseases. We will examine the main allopathic causes of fungal skin diseases in this chapter.

1. Fungal Pathogens:

Dermatophytes, a class of fungi that are particularly adept at infecting the skin, hair, and nails, are the main culprits behind fungus-related skin illnesses. The dermatophytes 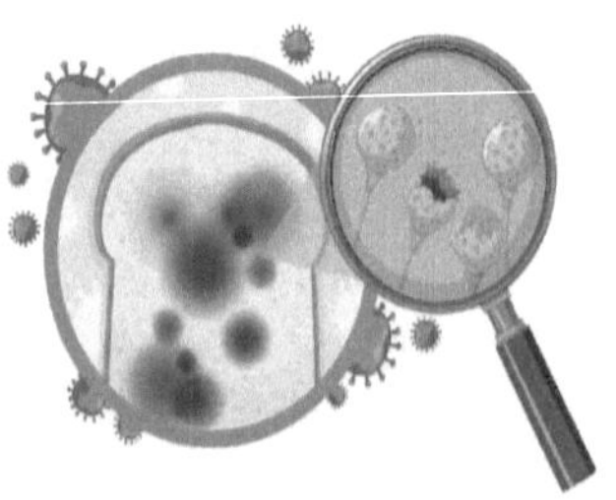 Trichophyton, Microsporum, and Epidermophyton species are frequently implicated in causing fungal skin infections. These fungi are extremely infectious and flourish in warm, humid settings.

2. Direct Connection:

Direct contact with an infected individual or contaminated objects is one of the most typical ways that fungal skin diseases are spread. Fungal spores can spread when personal objects like towels, clothes, or sporting goods are shared with an affected person.

3. Third-party Contact:

Another important factor contributing to fungal skin infections is indirect contact with contaminated surfaces or settings. People who go barefoot in public spaces like locker rooms, swimming pools, or shared showers may come into contact with fungal spores that are on the floors and carpets.

4. Microtrauma to the skin:

Microtrauma or minor skin wounds might serve as access sites for fungi. Fungi can enter the skin through scratches, scrapes, or places of friction, like the space between the toes.

5. Humid and Warm Climates:

Certain bodily parts are more prone to infection because fungi prefer warm, damp environments. Fungi thrive best in body creases, such as those seen in the groin, underarms, and areas between the toes.

6. Immune System Weakness:

Fungal skin infections are more common in those with compromised immune systems, such as those with HIV/AIDS, diabetes, or those receiving immunosuppressive therapies. A weakened immune system can find it difficult to establish a successful fight against fungi.

7. Prolonged Sweating:

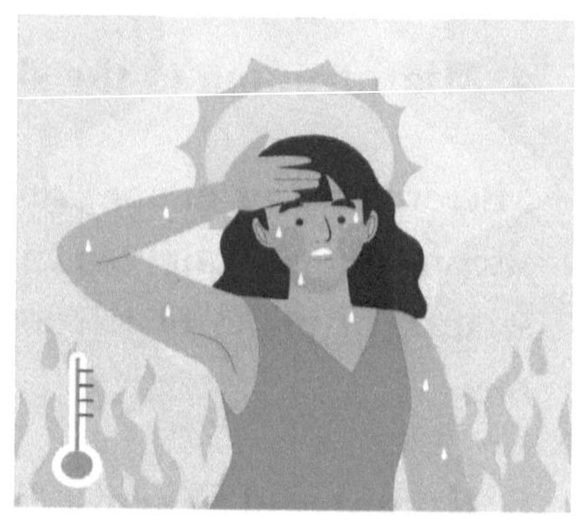

Over Sweating can provide a humid environment on the skin's surface that is more hospitable to the development of fungi. People who perspire a lot are more likely to get fungal skin infections, especially in places where moisture tends to collect.

8. Consistent Antibiotic Use:

Antibiotic usage for an extended period of time or often can change the balance of bacteria on the skin and mucous membranes. This instability might present a chance for fungus to flourish and spread illnesses.

9. Skin conditions you may already have:

The skin's natural barrier may be weakened by some underlying skin diseases like eczema or psoriasis, which makes it simpler for fungi to enter the body and spread infections.

10. Personal hygiene:

The spread of fungal skin infections can be facilitated by poor personal hygiene habits, such as infrequent handwashing and irregular bathing. To lower the risk of illness, proper cleanliness is crucial.

11. Close Personal Relationship:

The spread of fungal infections can be facilitated by close contact with an infected person, such as hugging or sharing a bed. It's possible for healthy skin to come into touch with fungal spores shed by the diseased person.

12. Dressing in Tight or Breathless Clothes:

Wearing clothing that is too tight or made of materials that are not permeable to moisture can trap moisture against the skin and foster the growth of fungi. Particularly in friction-prone environments, it is widespread.

In order to treat and prevent fungal skin infections, it is essential to understand their causes. To effectively treat fungal skin infections, allopathic medicine provides a variety of antifungal therapies, including topical and oral drugs. In order to stop the infection from spreading and creating discomfort, early diagnosis and treatment are crucial.

Despite so many possibilities for getting infected, it does not always happen, as we are protected by our skin barrier and local immune protection. Also the role of a healthy local skin microbiome is not very well studied so far in protecting from fungal skin infections.

Causes of fungal skin infection according to ayurveda-

The ancient Indian medical system known as Ayurveda offers a distinctive viewpoint on the origins of fungal skin infections, also known as "Dadru" or "Khadira" in Ayurvedic terminology. According to Ayurveda, imbalances in the body's doshas, notably Pitta and Kapha, are chiefly responsible for fungal skin infections and are brought on by a confluence of physiological, environmental, and lifestyle variables. According to Ayurvedic principles, we shall investigate the origins of fungal skin diseases in this chapter.

1. Dosha Imbalance:

The idea of doshas, the fundamental energy that controls the body, is a cornerstone of ayurveda. Skin infections caused by fungi are frequently linked to Pitta and Kapha dosha imbalances.

- **Pitta Imbalance:** The Pitta dosha can cause the body to overheat, which can cause inflammation, itchiness, and redness on the skin. The atmosphere that this extra heat might produce is conducive to the growth of fungi.

This literally may translate into more of the inflammatory presentations of the same fungus we see in different individuals, as the same fungal elements may present differently in different persons, when we see a pitta aggravation we may see more of an inflammatory presentation of tinea. If the principles of ayurvedic understanding are applied to this then the treatment outcomes are much better, this is my personal view and observation while treating hundreds of fungal infection patients.

- **Kapha Imbalance:** Imbalance in the Kapha dosha can cause dampness, coldness, and an excessive amount of moisture on the skin. Due to fungi's propensity for thriving in damp settings, these circumstances may facilitate fungal infections.

On the surface this explanation may sound a bit unscientific, but what a kapha avarana literally translates into in modern terms is a sluggishness of metabolism and maybe associated with a little unhealthy weight gain, once this happens and insulin resistance sets in there is perfect opportunity for fungal elements to thrive, thats why may patients with prediabetes and diabetes present to dermatology OPD with fungal infections.

2. Immune System Issues:

According to Ayurveda, a compromised immune system is a major contributor to the emergence of fungal skin diseases. A compromised immune system, or "Ojas," might increase a person's susceptibility to fungus and other external infections. Stress, a poor diet, and inactivity all have the potential to damage the immune system.

Again metabolic sluggishness may be the interpretation of the concept, leading up to slow brewing but chronic infections like fungal infections.

3. Poor Digestive Health:

Ama, or a buildup of toxins in the body, is a result of weak digestion, or "Mandagni" in Ayurvedic terminology. These toxins can harm the skin and circulate in the circulation, making it more prone to diseases, such as fungal skin infections.

4. Nutritional Factors:

Ayurveda places a high value on nutrition and how it affects general health. Eating meals that are directly at odds with one's dosha constitution or foods that are very hot, greasy, or difficult to digest can cause dosha imbalances, which can lead to skin problems like fungus infections.

5. Environmental Considerations:

Fungi may thrive on the skin when exposed to humid and moist environments, among other environmental variables. Protecting the skin from excessive moisture is advised by Ayurveda, especially in areas with high humidity.

6. Personal Hygiene:

Poor personal hygiene habits can cause perspiration, grime, and oil to build up on the skin's surface, which can foster the growth of fungi. To avoid skin diseases, Ayurveda places a strong emphasis on routine cleaning and preserving personal cleanliness.

7. Excessive use of chemicals and cosmetics:

Overuse of skincare products and cosmetics can upset the skin's natural balance and make it more vulnerable to fungus infections. The usage of natural and gentle skincare products is advised by ayurveda.

8. Emotional and Stress Factors:

The influence of emotional stress and mental health on the homeostasis of the body is acknowledged by Ayurveda, as is the mind-body link. High amounts of stress and emotional imbalances can upset the balance of the dosha, which can impair skin health and perhaps result in fungus infections.

9. Seasonal variables:

The effects of seasonal fluctuations on skin health are taken into account by ayurveda. The dosha balance can be upset by changing seasons, especially from the wet to the winter season, which can result in skin conditions like fungus infections.

It is crucial to comprehend these factors in the Ayurvedic context if one wants to effectively treat fungal skin diseases. In order to balance the doshas, boost the immune system, and maintain good hygiene, ayurvedic therapies for these illnesses frequently entail dietary changes, herbal medications, and lifestyle modifications.

To attain optimum skin health, Ayurveda promotes an individualized treatment strategy that works with each person's particular constitution and imbalances.

Besides the deeper concepts there are some oils which have a direct antifungal effect, there are some oils which have been shown to have antifungal properties, so when used as an adjuvant for treating fungal skin infections the results are superior and the need for oral antifungals is significantly reduced.

A series of more than 100 patients *treated without any oral antifungal medication with complete resolution and no recurrence noted after 6 months of treatment.*

The patients were all patients who had treatment failure or partial improvement of their fungal skin infections with previous recommended treatment with oral and topical antifungals.

Such patients were advised to apply a commonly used ayurvedic oil for 60-90 min before bath daily or apply daily once and keep on skin for 60-90 min then wash off. Followed by use of a conventional antifungal ciclopirox cream or eberconazole cream.

All patients were only concomitantly administered oral antihistamines on an as needed basis only, and were given oral multivitamin b , vitamin d and vitamin E supplements.

A remarkable improvement was seen in most patients, and almost all improved and completely recovered, 6 patients dropped out of the evaluation and could not be further contacted.

However the official publication and statistical evaluation has not been done. The observations do warrant a more detailed and elaborate evaluation to tackle the growing epidemic of fungal skin infections not just in India but around the world.

It is also important to note the recent reported discovery of a new species of fungus causing skin infections.

Questions to ask yourself if you have fungal skin infection

Dermatophytosis and tinea are other names for fungal skin diseases that can affect different parts of the body and take many different shapes. It's important to ask yourself a series of questions to better understand the variables causing your skin disease before pursuing particular therapies. These inquiries can assist you in determining possible causes and point you in the direction of practical remedies for treating and avoiding fungal skin diseases.

- **Have You Ever Had a Fungal Infection?** Take into account whether you have ever had a fungal skin illness because recurrence is frequently seen.

- **Do You Have Diabetes?** Consider your general health because several medical disorders, such as diabetes, might increase your risk of developing fungal skin infections. Is there a history of fungus infections in the family? Examine the frequency of fungal illnesses in your family, since genetics may contribute to susceptibility.

- **How Would You Describe Your Present Diet?** Examine your eating patterns because a diet rich in sugar and processed carbs might lead to fungus infections.

- **Do you have any more symptoms?** Keep track of any supplementary symptoms, such as scaling, redness, or itching, since they might reveal information about the kind of fungal infection.

- **What skincare items do you employ?** Check the ingredients in your skincare products, especially if they are excessively harsh or include irritants for your skin.

- **How Frequently Do You Shower or Bathe?** Examine your bathing practices because Bad hygiene might lead to fungal growth.

- **Do you properly dry your skin?** After a shower, pay attention to how well you dried your skin, especially in areas that were likely to retain moisture.

- **Are You Frequently in Moist Environments?** Consider your living circumstances and if you regularly enter moist or humid surroundings.

- **Do You Spend Time in Neighborhoods?** Think twice before using public restrooms, saunas, or swimming pools as these spaces might expose you to fungi.

- **Which Clothing Style Do You Wear?** Consider your wardrobe selections, especially if you wear clothing made of tight or impermeable materials that hold moisture against the skin.

- **What Kind of Shoes Do You Wear?** Consider your footwear options, especially if you wear footwear that prevents adequate airflow.

- **Do You Engage in Physical Activity or Sports?** Take into account if you participate in activities that need close physical contact since doing so may raise your chance of transmitting fungus.

- **Are You a Regular Swimmer or Workout Attendee?** If you often use gyms or swimming pools, be aware that these places may contain fungus spores.

- **How Frequently Do You Wash Your Feet and Hands?** Examine your foot and hand cleanliness because they are prone to fungus infections.

- **Do You Let Others Use Your Personal Items?** Think twice before sharing personal belongings with others, such as towels, razors, or shoes, as this might result in fungal infection.

- **Have You Been to a Tropical or Moist Area?** Take into account any recent trip to regions where fungal infections could be more common.

- **Do you currently have any skin conditions?** Keep an eye out for any underlying skin issues like psoriasis or eczema as they might undermine the skin's natural barrier.

These queries might help you get an important understanding of the possible root causes of your skin disease. Once you've determined the possible contributing causes, you may take specific action to better address and manage fungal skin infections. It's crucial to speak with a dermatologist or healthcare provider for a comprehensive assessment and advice tailored to your unique circumstances.

Treatment options for Fungal Skin Infection in Allopathy

Dermatophytosis, commonly referred to as tinea or fungal skin infections, are frequent dermatological disorders that can affect different parts of the body, such as the feet (athlete's foot), groin (jock itch), and body (ringworm). The conventional medical approach known as allopathy provides a variety of efficient management and eradication methods for fungal skin diseases. The major allopathic therapies for fungus-related skin infections will be discussed in this chapter.

1. Drugs with topical mycotoxins:

In order to treat fungal skin infections, topical antifungal creams, ointments, and powders are frequently the first line of treatment. They function by concentrating on and eliminating the fungi that are present on the skin's surface. These topical therapies 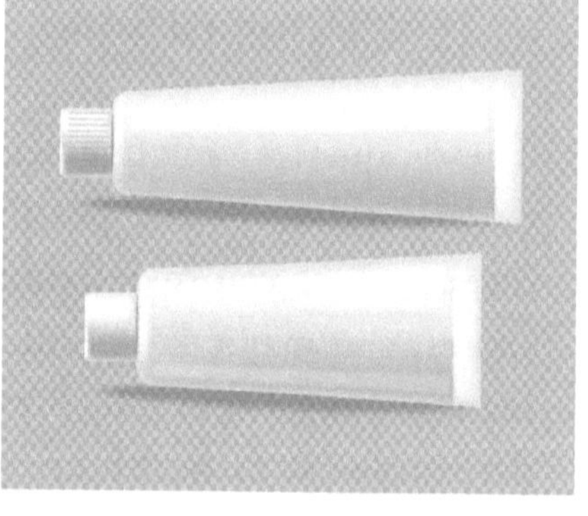 frequently employ the following antifungal substances:

- Clotrimazole
- Miconazole
- Terbinafine
- Ketoconazole
- Econazole
- Naftifine
- Butenafine

To guarantee total eradication of the infection, these over-the-counter and prescription drugs may need to be administered for many weeks and are often applied directly to the infected region.

2. Oral Antifungal medicines:

Oral antifungal medicines may be administered for fungal skin infections that are more severe or resistant. These oral treatments eradicate the fungus from the body systemically and are administered by mouth. Typical oral antifungal medications include:

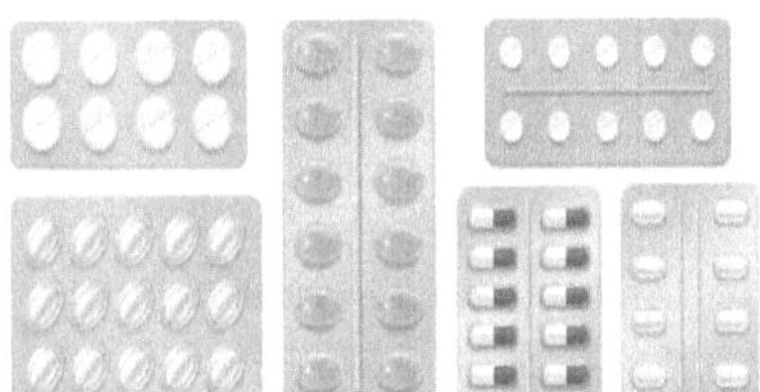

- Terbinafine
- Griseofulvin
- Fluconazole
- Itraconazole

The usage of oral antifungals should be properly supervised by a healthcare professional and is often recommended for a certain length of time.

3. Adjuvant Therapy:

In rare instances, a healthcare professional may suggest a mix of topical and oral antifungal medications to treat very difficult-to-treat or severe fungal skin infections. Combination therapy might offer a more thorough method of getting rid of the illness.

4. Creams with steroids (to treat inflammation):

Topical steroid creams may be recommended when a fungal skin infection causes considerable inflammation, redness, and itching. These lotions aid in reducing the pain and swelling brought on by the illness. Steroids should only be taken when prescribed by a doctor since, if misused, they might make the fungal infection worse.

5. Antifungal Shampoo:

Antifungal shampoos with chemicals like ketoconazole can be used to treat fungal skin diseases of the scalp, often known as tinea capitis. By using these shampoos often, you may get rid of fungal diseases on your scalp and hair.

6. Over-the-counter (OTC) Products:

For the treatment of fungal skin infections, a variety of over-the-counter (OTC) antifungal medications are readily accessible. Active chemicals like clotrimazole, miconazole, or terbinafine are frequently included in these products. While over-the-counter medicines can be helpful for minor infections, it is best to speak with a healthcare professional if the infection persists or becomes serious.

7. Maintaining Dry and Clean Skin:

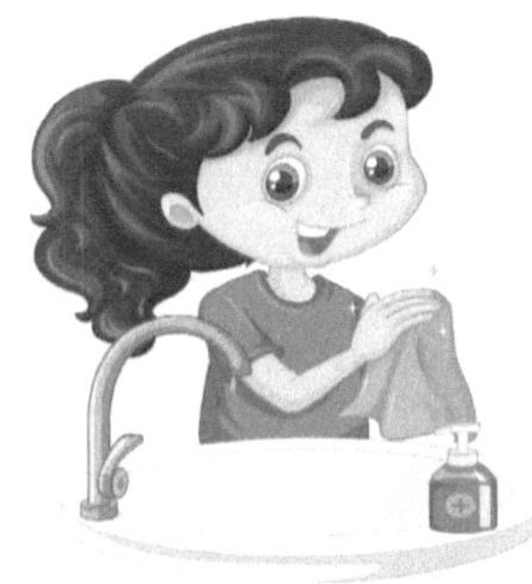

For the management and prevention of fungal skin infections, proper hygiene procedures are crucial, such as keeping the afflicted region dry and clean. Another way to maintain a dry atmosphere that is less conducive to fungal development is by using antifungal powders or sprays.

8. Prevention:

It's essential to stop fungal skin infections from returning. This entails practicing excellent personal hygiene, refraining from sharing personal belongings, dressing comfortably, and exercising caution in high-risk settings like swimming pools or locker rooms.

Note: For an accurate diagnosis and a treatment strategy customized for your unique illness, speak with a healthcare professional. Since fungus-related skin infections can occasionally resemble other skin problems, a proper diagnosis is necessary for efficient treatment.

In conclusion, allopathy offers a wide range of efficient treatment choices for fungus-related skin infections, including topical, oral, and combination therapies. These therapies, when used under the supervision of a healthcare professional, can aid in the eradication of the infection and offer relief from the discomfort and itching brought on by fungal skin disorders.

Integrative Medicine Approach to treat Fungal Skin Infections

Dermatophytosis and tinea, two common skin disorders that may be successfully treated with the Integrative Medical Approach, are caused by fungus. This all-encompassing strategy for health and wellbeing includes traditional medical procedures as well as alternative therapies, dietary changes, lifestyle alterations, and homeopathic cures. The Integrative Medical

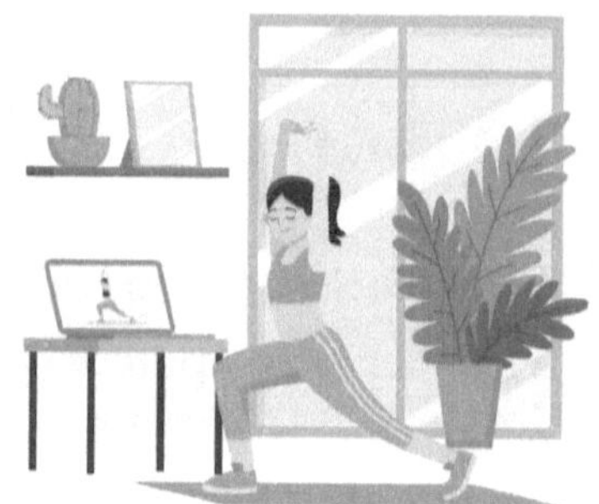

Approach offers a thorough plan to manage and treat disease by taking into account the interaction of several elements, including the body's intrinsic healing potential.

Integrative Approach to Understanding Fungal Skin Infections:

According to the Integrative Medical Approach, fungal skin diseases are the result of internal imbalances. These imbalances can be caused by a variety of circumstances, including reduced immunity, poor eating habits, stress, hormone cycles, and environmental impacts.

Rather than simply treating the outward symptoms, this method seeks to address the underlying causes in order to promote long-term healing and general well-being.

1. Immune System Aid:

A strong immune system is essential for avoiding and fighting fungal infections. The Integrative Medical Approach stresses immune system strengthening through dietary changes, exercise, and stress management. Nutrient-dense diets, frequent physical exercise, and stress-reduction strategies such as meditation or yoga can all help the body resist fungal infections.

2. Dietary Alterations:

Diet is critical in the treatment of fungal skin diseases. Individuals can lower their vulnerability to fungal overgrowth by identifying and eliminating probable dietary factors. Avoiding sweets, processed meals, and items that increase inflammation may be part of this. To boost gut health and immunity, integrative practitioners frequently advocate eating meals high in probiotics, prebiotics, and antioxidants.

3. Herbal and dietary supplements:

To strengthen the body's defenses against fungal infections, integrative medicine may use herbal medicines and nutritional supplements. To address the fundamental causes, natural antifungal medicines such as oregano oil, garlic, and grapefruit seed extract can be utilized in conjunction with dietary modifications.

4. Stress Management:

Stress can weaken the immune system and make fungal infections worse. Stress-reduction treatments such as mindfulness, meditation, acupuncture, and massage therapy are used in integrative therapies to reduce the influence of stress on the body's capacity to battle fungal overgrowth.

5. Hygiene and Skin Care:

In an Integrative Medical Approach, proper skin care and hygiene habits are critical. It is recommended that people keep the afflicted region clean and dry, and that they utilize natural, mild skin care products. Avoiding the usage of harsh

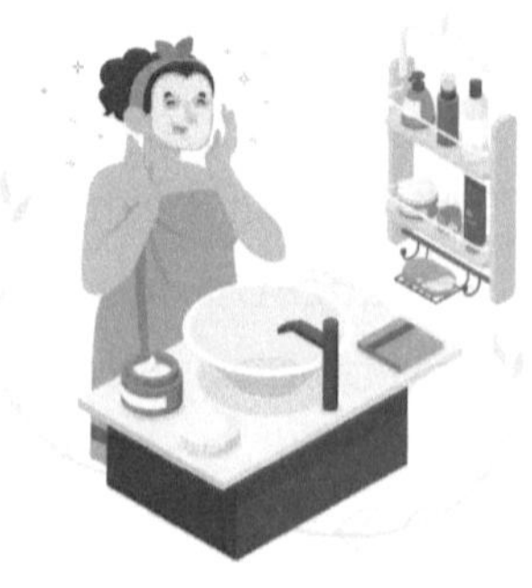

chemical-based cosmetics aids in the preservation of the skin's natural equilibrium.

6. Conventional Medicine:

Traditional therapies such as Ayurveda and Traditional Chinese Medicine (TCM) may be incorporated into the treatment plan, with the goal of restoring balance in the body's energies (doshas in Ayurveda, Qi in TCM). These ancient traditions frequently provide holistic treatments to fight fungal skin infections.

7. Customized Treatment Plans:

The Integrative Medical Approach emphasizes individualized treatment strategies. Practitioners personalize advice to treat particular underlying problems based on an individual's unique health history, dietary preferences, and lifestyle.

8. Preventative Actions:

An important component of this method is preventing the recurrence of fungal skin infections. Integrative practitioners advise patients on how to maintain appropriate personal cleanliness, food habits, and lifestyle choices in order to reduce the risk of recurring infections. Individuals can handle fungal skin infections holistically by combining the many aspects of the Integrative Medical Approach, addressing both the obvious symptoms and the underlying imbalances that lead to these illnesses. It's critical to work with integrative medicine experts to develop a specific treatment plan that fits your needs.

Pro tips to manage your fungal skin infections
  1) *Always seek a professional dermatology opinion*
  2) *Never use topical steroid creams , never more than 7-15 days, even if prescribed by your GP, talk to a derm.*

  3) *Wear natural fabrics*

  4) *Keep the washing machine disinfected, and dry it up at times.*
  5) *Do something to get your nutritional deficiencies evaluated and treated, the deficiencies are extremely important to launch an immune response to fungus.*
  6) *Avoid wearing dri-fit or synthetic fabrics.*

  7) *Keep the areas dry but the skin barrier should be well hydrated and skin barrier repair is important, you can use Cica creams from various brands or hydrocolloid gel creams for repair , also can add nano silver preparations to synergise anti fungal treatments.*
  8) *Adding a topical antifungal property laden oil before bath may be a good idea.*
  9) *Can consider some probiotic skin cream as a moisturizer, but effects are not very well studied.*

DANDRUFF:

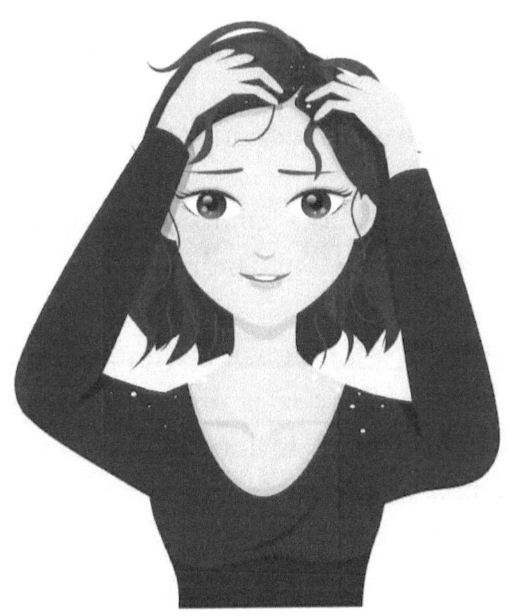

Understanding and Managing Dandruff: A Comprehensive Examination

Dandruff is a common and frequently irritating scalp ailment that affects people of all ages and backgrounds. It is distinguished by the shedding of white or gray flakes of dead skin from the scalp, which is accompanied by irritation and, in some cases, redness. Dandruff may be a cosmetic issue as well as a source of discomfort, so understanding its origins and effective treatment methods is critical. In this chapter, we'll look at dandruff from two different medical perspectives: allopathy and Ayurveda, discussing its origins, self-assessment questions, allopathic treatment choices, and an integrated dermatological strategy to effectively manage and prevent dandruff.

Dandruff Causes According to Allopathy:

The standard medical approach, allopathy, identifies various probable causes of dandruff:

1. Overgrowth of fungus: Overgrowth of a yeast-like fungus called Malassezia is one of the major causes of dandruff. This fungus is normally present on the scalp, but in certain people, it can multiply and cause dandruff. Malassezia overgrowth can cause scalp itching and flaking.

It is not just the overgrowth of the yeast but also one's immune response to the yeast, some body types react much to the yeast antigens and there is redness, itchiness and exfoliative reactions leading to the classical picture of dandruff.

2. Seborrheic Dermatitis: Seborrheic Dermatitis is a common skin disorder that causes redness, greasy or oily skin, and dandruff. It is assumed to be caused by an excess of sebum (skin oil) and is connected with Malassezia.

3. Dry Scalp: Dry skin on the scalp can cause flaking, which can be confused with dandruff. Dry scalp can be exacerbated by harsh weather, hot showers, or using shampoos that deplete natural oils.

Most shampoos can cause dryness as they are surfactant or detergent based. The quantity of shampoo, the frequency and the status of ones hormones all play a role in dryness of scalp, it is often confused with seborrheic dermatitis, where antifungals don't help and in some cases patients complain of burning or stinging sensation due to anti fungal shampoos or symptoms getting worse with use of antifungal shampoos. Many modern dermatologists do not recommend use of hair oil , and often dandruff patients have never oiled their scalp for months to years, which is considered a detrimental practice as per ayurveda.

4. Hair Care Product Sensitivity: Some people are sensitive to specific hair care products, such as shampoos, conditioners, or hair colors. These products might irritate the skin, resulting in dandruff-like symptoms.

5. Stress: Excessive stress can aggravate skin issues such as dandruff. Stress is thought to damage the immune system and might cause or aggravate dandruff symptoms.

Many patients note an aggravation of symptoms during stressors like exams or office presentations , appraisal and especially during travel, when diet is also impacted at such times.

6. Other Skin Conditions: Psoriasis and eczema, for example, can damage the scalp and cause dandruff-like symptoms.

Dandruff Causes According to Ayurveda:

Ayurveda, an ancient Indian medical tradition, provides a new viewpoint on the origins of dandruff. Ayurvedic practitioners believe that dandruff is caused by an imbalance in the doshas, or the body's innate energies:

1. Vata Imbalance: Dandruff can be caused by a Vata dosha imbalance, which is characterized by dryness. Vata oversees the components of air and ether, and when irritated, it can cause a dry, flaky scalp.

Use of medicated oils and soaking the scalp , head and neck in oil is of paramount importance in vata imbalance related dandruff

2. Kapha Imbalance: An overabundance of the Kapha dosha, which represents water and earth components, can also lead to dandruff. Dandruff that is greasy, oily, and sticky might indicate a Kapha imbalance.

Such type of dandruff may be accompanied by "kleda" or dermal edema, kind of peau d'orange appearance, such patients MAY NOT BENEFIT FROM OILING THERAPIES, THIS IS HOW AYURVEDA DIFFERENTIATES REGARDING PERSONALIZED , INDIVIDUALISED TREATMENT EVEN IN CASE OF TRIVIAL CONCERNS LIKE DANDRUFF.

3. Poor nutrition and Digestion: Ayurveda emphasizes the relationship between nutrition and skin health.

Excessive consumption of cold, heavy, or processed meals might affect digestion, resulting in dandruff.

4. Stress and Emotional Factors: Ayurveda, like allopathy, recognizes the impact of stress on dandruff. Stress can disrupt the dosha balance, impacting skin health and potentially leading to dandruff.

5. Improper Hair Care: Ayurveda emphasizes the need of good hair care on a regular basis. Dandruff can be exacerbated by using harsh shampoos, overwashing the hair, and ignoring oil massages.

Questions to Consider If You Have Dandruff:

Understanding the possible reasons of your dandruff entails asking yourself the following questions:

1. Have you noticed any redness or itchiness? Dandruff is frequently associated with redness and itching. Determine whether you are suffering any of these symptoms.

2. Is the dandruff dry or oily? Take into account the look and texture of your dandruff. Dry dandruff may suggest a Vata imbalance, but oily dandruff may indicate a Kapha imbalance.

3. Is Stress a Problem in Your Life? Consider your stress levels as well as any recent stressful situations. Stress may be a major cause of dandruff.

4. Do You Eat a Well-Balanced Diet? Examine your eating habits to see if they are consistent with Ayurvedic principles. A dosha-balancing diet can help avoid dandruff.

5. Are You Using the Correct Hair Care Routine? Examine your hair-care routine. Make certain that it includes gentle washes, oil massages, and adequate hydration.

6. Have You Had Any Digestive Problems? According to Ayurveda, digestive issues such as bloating or indigestion might be caused by dandruff.

7. Have You Noticed Any Seasonal Changes? Seasonal changes might have an effect on dandruff. Ayurveda studies how the seasons affect dosha balance, which can affect skin.

8. Do you use hair care products on a regular basis? Examine your hair care items, including shampoos, conditioners, and style aids. Some substances may cause scalp irritation.

Allopathic Treatment Options:

Allopathy provides several dandruff treatment options:

1. Antifungal Shampoos: Antifungal shampoos, such as ketoconazole or selenium sulfide, can help treat Malassezia overgrowth.

The newer luliconazole shampoos may help some resistant fungal patients. Also some preparations are there with salicylic acid and antifungal together, such preparations may be best suited for patients with oily scalp and crusty dandruff. But incase of oozing and redness of the scalp, there may be a stinging sensation with salicylic acid preparations.

2. Tar-Based Shampoos: Shampoos containing coal tar help relieve itching and flaking by slowing the proliferation of skin cells on the scalp.

Such preparations often are accompanied by patient perception of dryness of scalp and thinning of hair, most conventional cheaper preparations may make the hair dry and frizzy, there are some preparations which come with conditioners and may be better tolerated. Also prolonged use of tar on the scalp is not recommended for risk of possibility of long term side effects.

3. Salicylic Acid Shampoos: Salicylic acid shampoos are helpful in breaking down flakes and removing them from the scalp. They can efficiently manage dandruff.

- ***Zinc pyrithione shampoos:*** Shampoos containing zinc pyrithione function by slowing down the formation of skin cells, which is commonly enhanced in people with dandruff.

- ***Corticosteroid Lotions:*** Corticosteroid lotions or creams may be recommended in severe situations to relieve inflammation and irritation on the scalp. However, because of the possibility of negative effects, they should only be taken under medical supervision and for a limited time.

There are clobetasol and fluocinonide shampoos available but should definitely not be used for too long.

- ***Prescription drugs:*** When other treatments fail, a doctor may prescribe oral antifungal drugs or antibiotics to treat severe dandruff problems.

Dandruff Treatment Using an Integrated Dermatology Approach:

For successful dandruff control, the integrated dermatological approach combines conventional treatments with alternative therapies, dietary changes, and lifestyle changes. This method can be used as follows: Ayurvedic beliefs emphasize the importance of eating a well-balanced diet. Include meals that will help to balance your doshas, such as warming foods for Vata and light, non-greasy foods for Kapha. Foods high in omega-3 fatty acids, antioxidants, and vitamins can also help keep your scalp healthy.

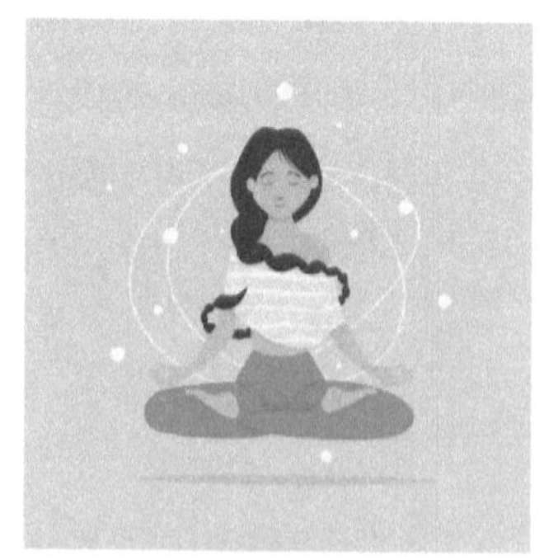

1. Stress Management: Incorporate stress-reduction practices such as meditation, yoga, or deep breathing exercises into your regular routine. Stress reduction is critical for dandruff management, especially when Vata or emotional stresses are present.

2. Herbal and nutritional supplements: Some herbal remedies and nutritional supplements can be used in addition to or instead of conventional therapies. Natural anti-inflammatory and antifungal qualities of neem and aloe vera, for example, may help calm the scalp.

3. Proper Hair Care: Establish a hair care regimen that promotes scalp health. Use moderate, natural shampoos and refrain from overwashing. Ayurvedic therapies such as warm oil scalp massages can enhance circulation and moisturize the scalp.

4. Dietary Changes: Avoid dietary factors that aggravate dandruff. If you've discovered that certain foods aggravate your symptoms, consider removing or limiting them from your diet.

5. Individualized Care: The integrated dermatological approach offers tailored treatment strategies. Dermatologists offer treatment techniques based on an individual's unique health history, dosha imbalances, and lifestyle decisions.

6.Preventive Measures:

Managing dandruff entails not just treating it but also preventing recurrence. Integrative dermatologists advise patients on how to maintain appropriate 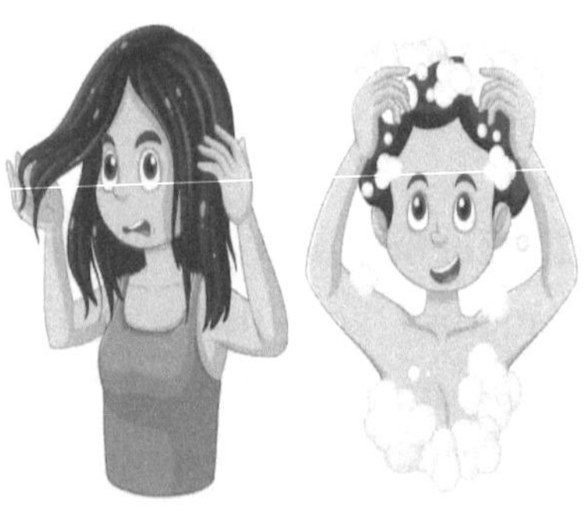 personal cleanliness, dietary habits, and lifestyle choices to reduce the risk of repeat dandruff episodes.

In conclusion, dandruff is a common problem for many people, and the causes are many. While allopathy provides effective therapy for symptoms, the integrated dermatological approach combines conventional therapeutics with Ayurvedic principles, dietary changes, and stress management to address both visible symptoms and underlying imbalances. It is critical to engage with healthcare experts who are familiar with this integrated approach in order to develop a personalized treatment plan that is tailored to your specific requirements and circumstances. Effective dandruff management can result in a healthier, more pleasant scalp and increased overall well-being.

Pro tips for Integrated dandruff management
1) Take care of nutritional deficiencies especially mineral and micro mineral deficiencies, calcium, magnesium, copper, zinc, selenium, chromium, iron etc.
2) Vitamin d, E, B, deficiencies may also play an important role.
3) It is best to take natural origin supplements in adequate dose especially if absorption is compromised or if dietary intake is not enough

4) I would personally always recommend using an good ayurvedic oil, some have been evaluated for topical antifungal activity, like sidda oils with hibiscus , neem and other extracts in a base of coconut oil
5) Minimize use of oral antifungals- but when needed stick to recommended dose and durations as per current local guidelines
6) Try going on a completed detox diet for 30-40 days, comprising complete abstinence from all caffeinated foods, sugar, and all refined flour and processed foods. Also for some individuals in my practice we have noted an aggravation of symptoms with tea and coffee intake, same goes for carbonated, sugary beverages.

CHAPTER 12- PCOS And Hormonal Concerns

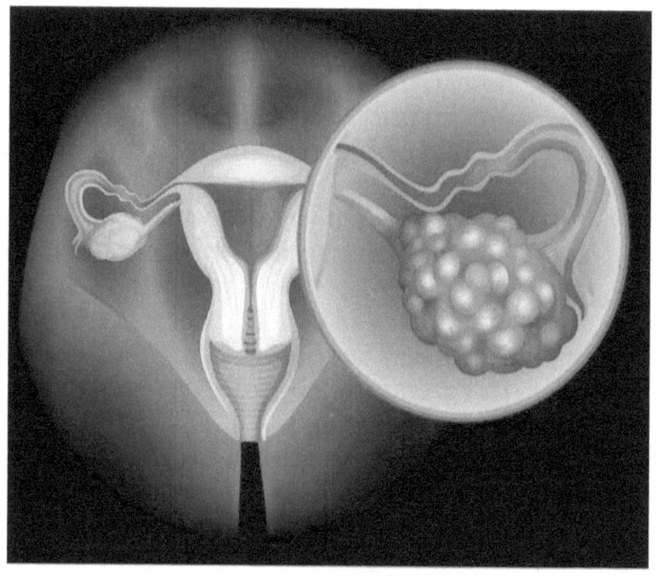

Causes of PCOS according to allopathy:

PCOS is a complicated endocrine disease that affects millions of women throughout the world. It is distinguished by a number of symptoms, including irregular menstrual cycles, increased androgens (male hormones), and the development of tiny cysts on the ovaries. While the precise origins of PCOS are unknown, allopathic medicine, often known as Western medicine, has made tremendous progress in identifying the components that contribute to this disorder.

Hormonal Imbalance:

PCOS is largely a hormonal condition. Normal endocrine system function is critical for the control of several body activities, including menstruation and ovulation. In women with PCOS, there is an imbalance of hormones, including insulin and sex hormones like estrogen and progesterone.

a. Insulin Resistance: Insulin resistance is a major role in the development of PCOS. Insulin is a hormone generated by the pancreas that aids in blood sugar regulation. Insulin resistance occurs when the body's cells do not respond adequately to insulin, resulting in greater amounts of insulin in the circulation. Excess insulin can cause the ovaries to generate more androgens like testosterone. Increased testosterone levels can interrupt the normal menstrual cycle, resulting in irregular or nonexistent periods.

b. Excess Androgen: Androgens are commonly thought to be masculine hormones, yet they are present in both men and women, albeit in varying amounts. Women with PCOS have an overabundance of androgens, which causes symptoms such as acne, hirsutism (excessive hair growth), and male-pattern baldness. High androgen levels can also interfere with ovarian follicle growth, resulting in the distinctive cysts observed on the ovaries in PCOS.

c. Estrogen and progesterone dysregulation: Estrogen and progesterone are the two principal female sex hormones that regulate the menstrual cycle and keep the reproductive system healthy. The ratio of these hormones is frequently out of balance in PCOS. Insulin resistance and increased androgens can affect estrogen and progesterone release and function. This can cause irregular or anovulatory (lack of ovulation) periods, both of which are typical symptoms of PCOS.

Genetic Variables

PCOS development is also influenced by genetic factors. According to research, women who have a family history of PCOS are more likely to get the disorder themselves. While particular genes linked to PCOS have yet to be found, it is evident that genetics can impact a person's susceptibility to the disorder.

Environmental Aspects

Lifestyle and nutritional decisions, for example, can contribute to the development and worsening of PCOS. Obesity, poor food habits, and a lack of physical activity have all been linked to an increased risk of insulin resistance and hormonal imbalances. A healthy lifestyle that includes a balanced diet and frequent exercise can help control PCOS symptoms and lessen its long-term consequences.

Inflammation:

Another possible cause of PCOS is chronic low-grade inflammation. Inflammation can cause insulin resistance and interfere with hormonal homeostasis. Obesity, which is frequently related with PCOS, is a well-documented cause of chronic inflammation. In certain circumstances, reducing inflammation through lifestyle modifications and drugs might help reduce PCOS symptoms.

Other Considerations

Other variables that might contribute to PCOS include:
- *Stress:* High amounts of stress can aggravate hormonal imbalances and worsen PCOS symptoms.
- ***Exposure to Endocrine-Disrupting substances:*** Endocrine disruptors are substances prevalent in the environment that might interfere with the normal function of hormones and potentially contribute to PCOS.

- ***Hypersecretion of Luteinizing Hormone (LH):*** Elevated levels of LH, a pituitary gland hormone, can disturb normal ovarian function and contribute to the development of PCOS.

To summarize, PCOS is a complicated illness with several contributing causes. Hormonal imbalances, insulin resistance, heredity, environmental factors, inflammation, and other factors all contribute to the onset of this illness. Allopathic treatment seeks to manage PCOS with a mix of lifestyle modifications, medication, and, in some cases, surgical procedures, treating the underlying reasons and easing the symptoms that women with PCOS suffer.

PRO TIPS ABOUT PCOS

Pcos either lean type of obese type with metabolic imbalance is a complex interplay of basically 3 types of hormones, to put it simply, these are insulin (food and fasting related), Stress hormone that is cortisol, (emotional states, chronic stressors etc.) and female steroid hormones the estrogens and progesterone metabolites.

1)It is extremely important to factor in the role of emotions, as if there are feelings of supression, anger, anxiety due to any reason, or any root cause of such psycho-emotional factors then these will trigger hormonal changes in due course of time.

2) Sleep wake cycle governs the circadian rhythm, the circadian rhythm inturn slowly but surely impacts thyroid and other female hormones impacting the regularity and flow of periods (28).

3) The role of foods affecting Metabolism especially dairy, cannot be neglected.

4) sugar may be adding to low grade inflammation and gut microbiome dysbiosis and thereby indirectly affecting the balance of hormones.

5) Abstinence from incriminating foods completely for a duration of time may assist in symptom reversal

6) If there are any digestive complaints like bloating, indigestion, irritable bowel or dysmotility type of symptoms, constipation etc all need active and energetic addressal for best management of pcos, just taking hormones for symptomatic improvement and for regularizing cycles may not work for all , and may not be the best option if used alone.

Causes of PCOS according to Ayurveda

Ayurveda, an ancient Indian system of traditional medicine, provides a comprehensive approach to addressing the origins of PCOS and associated hormonal issues. As major elements in the development and management of PCOS, Ayurveda emphasizes the balance of doshas (biological energies), lifestyle, food, and general well-being.

Imbalance of the Doshas:

According to Ayurveda, PCOS is caused by an imbalance in the doshas, particularly the Vata and Kapha doshas.

a. Imbalance of Vata Dosha: The Vata dosha governs mobility and circulation throughout the body. An overabundance of Vata energy might interfere with the regular functioning of the reproductive system. This imbalance may result in irregular menstruation and impaired ovulation, both of which are frequent symptoms of PCOS. Vata imbalances can be exacerbated by stress, unpredictable daily routines, and an unhealthy lifestyle.

In particular in ayurveda the role of Apana Vayu is paramount in concerns such as pcos and endometriosis. This force governs the eliminatory function of the lower abdomen and pelvis area.

b. Imbalance of the Kapha Dosha: The Kapha dosha is related to stability and sustenance. An overabundance of Kapha can cause mucus and fluids to build up in the body, potentially harming the ovaries. Because Kapha is involved in metabolism, this imbalance in PCOS can result in the production of cysts on the ovaries and insulin resistance. Poor nutrition, sedentary habits, and an abundance of sugary, greasy, and cold foods are said to aggravate Kapha dosha.

This also reflects in symptoms such as congestion and fluid retention and edema, the lymphatic circulation also gets affected which is very often neglected , poorly understood and least talked about in western medicine.

Impairment of Agni (Digestive Fire)

The potency of Agni, the digestive fire, is highly valued in Ayurveda. When Agni is weak or hindered, pollutants accumulate in the body, exacerbating dosha imbalances and damaging the hormonal system. Obesity and insulin resistance, both of which are frequent in PCOS, can be exacerbated by poor digestion.

Accumulation of Ama (Toxins)

According to Ayurveda, the buildup of Ama, or poisons, is a crucial cause in the development of PCOS. These poisons can clog the body's pathways, causing hormonal abnormalities and cyst growth in the ovaries. Ama is frequently caused by poor dietary choices, such as eating processed, heavy, and difficult-to-digest meals.

Poor Lifestyle Habits

Ayurveda places a high value on one's lifestyle and daily routine. Unhealthy lifestyle choices, such as irregular sleeping habits, a lack of exercise, and excessive stress, can upset the natural balance of doshas, impede Agni, and encourage Ama buildup. All of these variables have a role in the development and evolution of PCOS.

Emotional and psychological aspects

Ayurveda recognizes the link between emotional well-being and physical health. Emotional stress, worry, and unresolved emotional difficulties are thought to have an effect on the hormonal system, perhaps exacerbating PCOS symptoms. Meditation, yoga, and relaxation practices are advised for dealing with these emotional concerns.

Dietary Concerns

Diet is very important in Ayurveda. It is critical to consume meals that are compatible with a person's constitution (Prakriti) and to resolve any present imbalances. Ayurveda recommends a warm, light, and easily digested diet for PCOS, with an emphasis on whole grains, fresh fruits and vegetables, and herbal teas. It is also advised to limit or avoid processed and sugary meals.

Ultimately, Ayurveda provides a distinct viewpoint on the causes of PCOS and associated hormonal issues. It emphasizes dosha balance, digestive fire, toxin buildup, lifestyle choices, emotional variables, and dietary habits as interrelated elements impacting PCOS development. To restore balance and ease the symptoms of PCOS, Ayurvedic therapies often incorporate individualized techniques such as dietary adjustments, herbal medicines, yoga, meditation, and lifestyle changes.

It gets complex when it comes to diet and we see many divergent views when it comes to diet guidelines. Even amongst dermatologists and gynecologists the views are divergent. For example the opinions are divided about dairy and meat based diets, and sometimes even about the effects of soy.
I will try to give some clarity on these here

1) *The metabolism of different foods varies from individual to individual very widely*
2) *The same food may be working well for you for years and due to change in some factors like season, the combination how the food is taken, age etc may influence the adverse effects of food. For example there are patients who tolerate dairy all their life well but after a certain age develop intolerance to it, and the same people may be able to tolerate dairy again after quitting it for a duration of time.*

3) *The intake of preservative laden, ultra processed foods will change the way our microbiome behaves, and this will impact not just absorption of nutrients but may influence hormones also.(29) (30)*
4) *The newer food allergy tests and the gut microbiome studies may assist in finding out which foods may be suitable, but following an ayurvedic approach to DIET AS PER BODY TYPE AND AVOIDANCE OF FOOD COMBINATIONS AS PER SEASON, AGE AND INDIVIDUAL AYURVEDIC BODY TYPE ARE IMPORTANT, MOST PRACTICAL AND EFFECTIVE*

Questions to ask yourself if you have PCOS

Polycystic Ovary Syndrome (PCOS) is a complicated hormonal condition that affects women. It frequently manifests with a wide range of symptoms and health issues. Posing specific questions to yourself will help you understand the probable signs and symptoms of PCOS and their significance in directing your road to diagnosis and therapy.

Reproductive and Menstrual Health:

Are your menstrual cycles erratic, with periods that vary in length and timing?
Irregular periods are a defining feature of PCOS. This question assists you in identifying a common symptom of the illness. Menstrual cycles that are irregular might impact fertility and signal hormonal abnormalities.

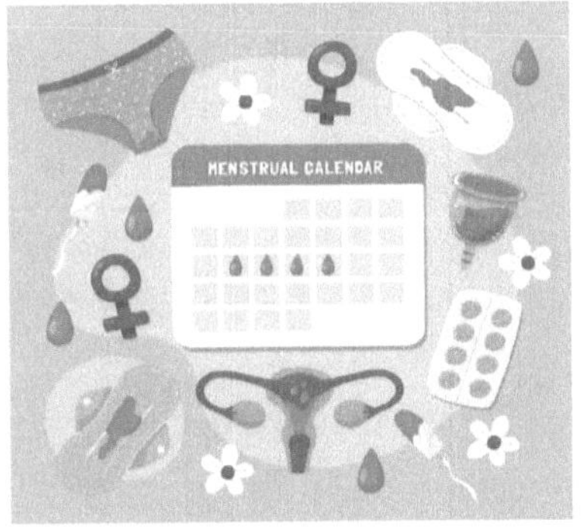

Do you have abnormally heavy or protracted menstrual bleeding?

Another typical symptom of PCOS is heavy and extended menstrual flow. It can cause anemia and have a detrimental influence on your quality of life.

Have you ever skipped a period or gone months without menstruating?

Amenorrhea, or the lack of periods, is a cause for concern since it indicates irregular ovulation. Understanding your menstrual history is critical for PCOS diagnosis.

Do you suffer from significant menstruation pain, such as cramping?

Menstrual discomfort can accompany PCOS and is often caused by abnormal hormone levels. It is critical to know if you have this symptom in order to make an accurate diagnosis.

Have you struggled to conceive or dealt with infertility?

Because of ovulatory issues, many people with PCOS are concerned about infertility. This question is crucial if you're attempting to conceive and having difficulties.

Do you have any odd hair growth on your face, chest, or back?

Hirsutism, or excessive hair growth in male-pattern regions, is a frequent symptom of PCOS caused by increased androgens. It is a critical diagnostic indication.

Physical Signs and Symptoms:

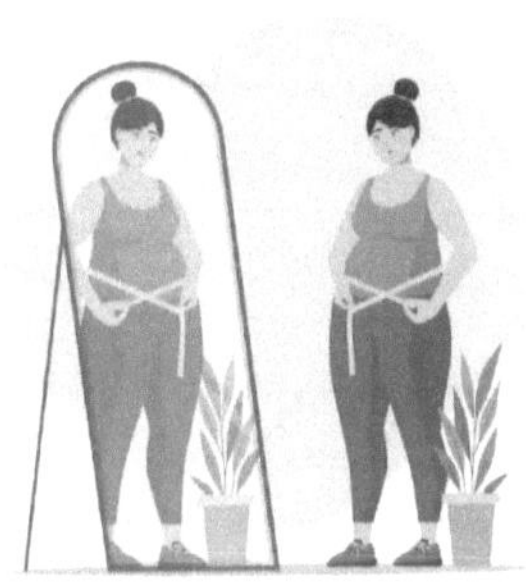

Have you seen unexpected weight gain, particularly around your abdomen?

Weight gain and problems reducing weight are prevalent in people with PCOS. Insulin resistance, a common problem in PCOS, is linked to abdominal fat formation.

Have you noticed hair thinning or loss, particularly on your scalp?

Thinning hair, or male-pattern baldness, is associated with increased androgens and is commonly noticed in PCOS.

Do you have dark skin spots, particularly in body folds such as the neck, armpits, or groin?

The patches, known as acanthosis nigricans, can be a symptom of insulin resistance, which is frequent in PCOS.

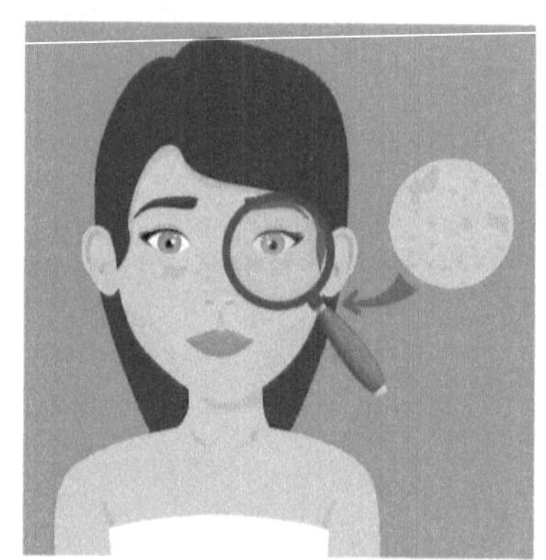

Is your skin prone to acne or has recurring breakouts?

Acne is frequently connected to hormonal abnormalities, which are a feature of PCOS.

Have you seen any tiny, painless cysts or nodules on your skin, especially around your neck or underarms?

These skin alterations, known as skin tags or acrochordons, are occasionally linked to insulin resistance, which is common in PCOS.

How has your sleep pattern been ? Do you sleep inadequately in terms of quality or quantity of sleep more than 2 days per week?

Do you often find yourself anxious and uncontrollably worrying more than 2 times per week?

Lifestyle and Health Habits:

Are your eating habits dominated by processed and high-sugar foods?

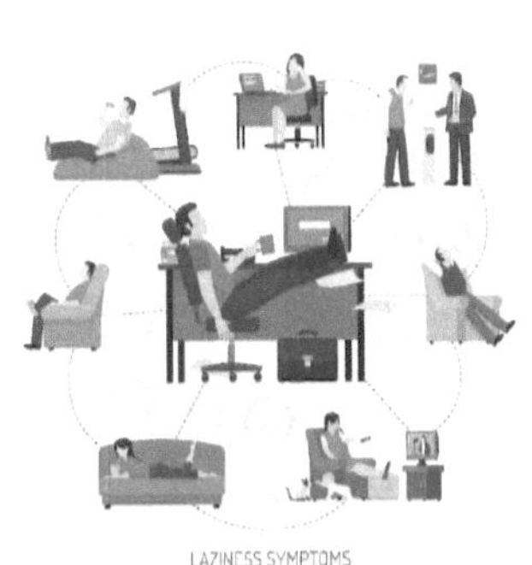

Poor food choices can aggravate insulin resistance and weight gain, which can exacerbate PCOS symptoms.

Do you live a sedentary lifestyle with little physical activity?
Sedentism can increase insulin resistance, weight gain, and general health in those with PCOS.

Have you been stressed out recently, or do you suffer from persistent anxiety or depression?
Stress can aggravate hormonal irregularities in PCOS, affecting both physical and mental health.

Have you been exercising moderately or no exercise at all? Have you been exercising too aggressively to lose weight or to maintain weight, especially exercising when mentally very stressed or sleep deprived?

Is there a family history of PCOS or other hormonal disorders?

Having a family history of PCOS increases your chances of having the disorder. Genetic factors influence its growth.

Medical and Gynecological History:

Have you been told you have insulin resistance or prediabetes?
Insulin resistance is frequently related with PCOS, and controlling it is critical for symptom management.

Have you ever been diagnosed with another hormonal illness, such as thyroid problems?
Other hormonal problems can coexist with PCOS and must be addressed for general health.

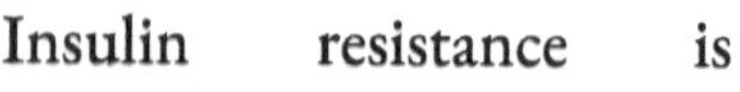

It may be a good idea to investigate not just for thyroid hormones but also for anti thyroid antibodies.

Have you undergone a pelvic ultrasound or any other diagnostic testing that detected ovarian cysts?
Pelvic ultrasonography is an important diagnostic technique for PCOS. Detecting cysts on the ovaries can help confirm a diagnosis.

It is highly recommended to specifically ask your radiologist to comment on the quality of OVARIAN STROMA when looking at the ultrasound of the lower abdomen, this significantly helps the gynae or treating physician make specific decisions.

Do your menstrual cycle cause mood swings, irritation, or emotional disturbances?

Hormonal imbalances can have an impact on mood, and recognizing these symptoms can aid in diagnosis and treatment.

Are you presently taking PCOS drugs or hormonal birth control to treat your symptoms?

Medications and birth control are frequently used to treat PCOS. It's critical to know whether you're presently undergoing any therapies.

Concerns About Long-Term Health:

Are you aware of the long-term health hazards connected with PCOS, such as an increased risk of diabetes, heart disease, or endometrial cancer?

Understanding the long-term health concerns linked with PCOS is critical for making educated health decisions.

Have you discussed your PCOS diagnosis with a healthcare practitioner and received treatment advice?
Seeking expert advice is critical for properly controlling PCOS and meeting your individual requirements.

Conclusion

If you suspect you have PCOS, these questions might help you begin your self-evaluation and reflection. Keep in mind that PCOS symptoms might vary greatly between people. If you answered yes to several of these questions, you should see a doctor, preferably a gynecologist or endocrinologist, for a full examination and tailored treatment plan. When living with PCOS, early diagnosis and care are critical to maintaining your health and well-being.

Treatment options for PCOS in Allopathy

Polycystic Ovary Syndrome (PCOS) is a complicated endocrine condition that necessitates a varied therapeutic strategy. Traditional allopathic treatment provides a variety of therapy alternatives for controlling PCOS symptoms and correcting the underlying hormonal abnormalities. The therapy chosen is determined by the individual's personal requirements and goals, as well as the severity of their ailment.

Changes in Lifestyle:

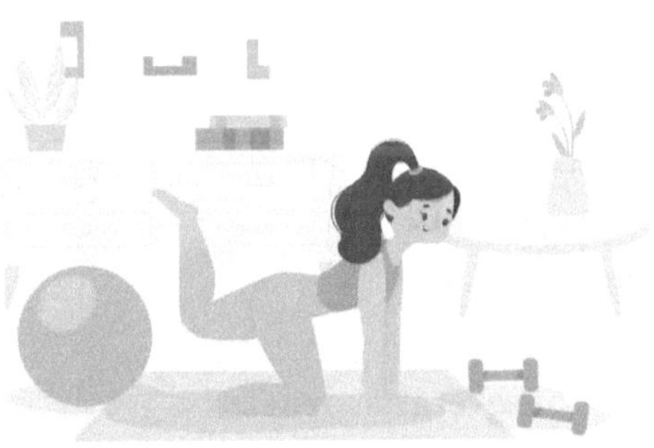

In addressing PCOS, lifestyle modifications are frequently the first line of defense. These changes can enhance general health and lessen the severity of symptoms.

- ***Dietary Changes:*** A well-balanced diet rich in complex carbs, fiber, and lean protein can help manage blood sugar levels. Reduced consumption of high-glycemic index foods and added sugars is essential for treating insulin resistance, which is frequent in PCOS.

- ***Exercise:*** Physical exercise is vital for weight management, increasing insulin sensitivity, and lowering the risk of obesity-related comorbidities. Typically, a mix of aerobic and strength-training workouts is advised.

- ***Weight Control:*** Achieving and maintaining a healthy weight is a fundamental objective in PCOS management. Even minor weight reduction can enhance menstrual regularity, fertility, and insulin sensitivity significantly.

Medicines:

There are several drugs available to treat the hormonal abnormalities and symptoms of PCOS.

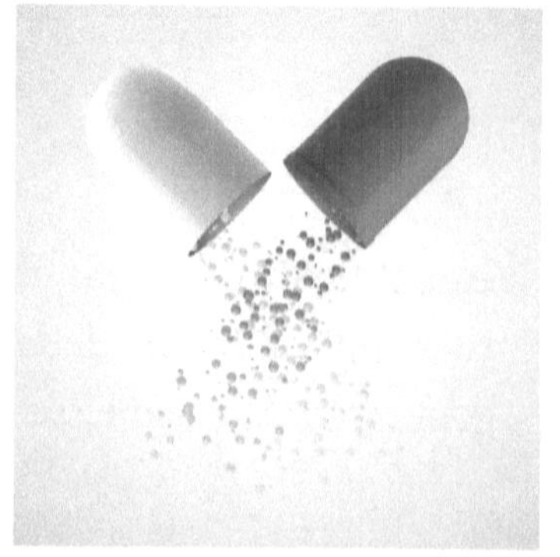

- ***Birth Control Pills:*** Birth control pills can

help regulate menstrual periods and lessen PCOS symptoms such as acne and excessive hair growth. They function by preventing the ovaries from producing androgens.

Taking OCP or birth control pills alone and not tackling the real root causes like exercise and food as per body type may not be a great choice towards holistic health practices.

- *Anti-Androgen Medications:* Anti-androgen medications such as spironolactone and finasteride may be used to treat excess hair growth (hirsutism) and acne. These drugs serve to mitigate the consequences of high androgen levels.

  Many medicines are available most commonly spironolactone and flutamide , bicalutamide are available , all of them come with some undesirable effects, such drugs must always be consumed under endocrinologist supervision and for a duration only as recommended.

- *Metformin:* Originally used to treat type 2 diabetes, metformin is now being utilized to treat insulin resistance in PCOS patients. It can aid in the regulation of menstrual periods and lower the chance of acquiring diabetes.

  This works really well for obese types of pcos, as this assists in ways more than one by insulin sensitizing it helps in many other ways. It is important to note here the role of fasting in helping insulin resistance.

- ***Clomiphene Citrate or Letrozole:*** These drugs are used to trigger ovulation in PCOS women who are attempting to conceive. They cause the ovaries to produce eggs.

- ***Gonadotropins:*** When oral drugs fail to trigger ovulation, injectable hormones such as FSH and hCG are employed.

Surgical Procedures:

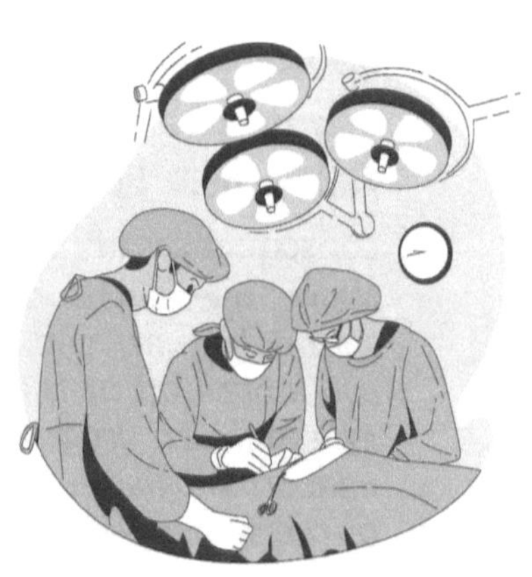

- ***Ovarian Drilling:*** If drugs and lifestyle changes have not resulted in ovulation, laparoscopic ovarian drilling can be done. To promote ovulation, tiny holes are made in the ovaries.

- ***Cyst Removal:*** When big ovarian cysts cause substantial pain or discomfort, surgical removal may be explored; however, this does not cure PCOS and is usually used as a last option.

Fertility Treatments:

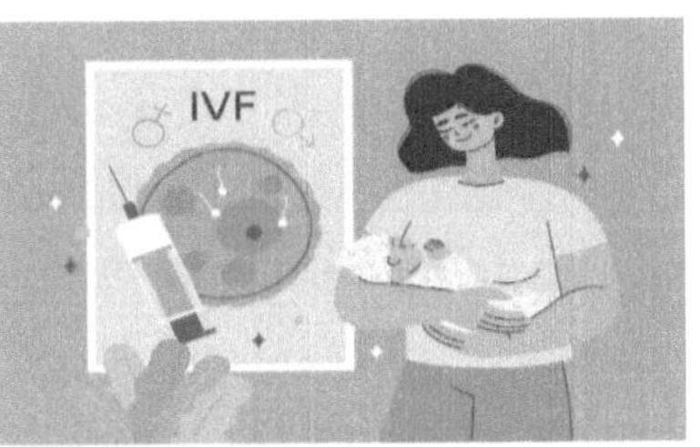

In Vitro Fertilization (IVF): For those with PCOS who are having difficulty conceiving, IVF may be advised. This method of assisted reproduction entails extracting eggs, fertilizing them in a laboratory, and implanting embryos in the uterus.

Symptom-Specific Care:

- ***Acne Treatment:*** Antibiotics and retinoids, as well as topical or oral medicines, can help treat acne symptoms.

- ***Hirsutism Management:*** Methods such as electrolysis, laser hair removal, or shaving, in conjunction to anti-androgen medicines, can help reduce unwanted hair development.

- ***Endometrial Protection:*** Progestin treatment may be administered to lower the risk of endometrial cancer in women who have irregular or missing menstrual periods.

Long-Term Health Care Management:

Diabetes and Cardiovascular Risk Management: Individuals with PCOS must regularly test their blood sugar levels and lipid profiles. Diabetes and cardiovascular disease can be reduced by lifestyle modifications, medicines, and weight control.

PCOS therapy is very unique, and it is critical that patients collaborate closely with a healthcare professional to build a specific treatment strategy. Regular follow-up sessions are required to assess progress and make any modifications to the treatment plan. PCOS can be successfully controlled, allowing people to live healthy and meaningful lives. PCOS symptoms can be reduced and long-term health concerns reduced with the correct therapy.

Integrated medical approach to treat PCOS

Polycystic Ovary Syndrome (PCOS) is a complicated endocrine condition characterized by a wide variety of symptoms affecting many bodily systems. To treat PCOS, an integrated medicine approach combines standard Western allopathic medication with complementary and alternative therapies. This method seeks to treat not just the symptoms of PCOS, but also the underlying reasons and the general well-being of those suffering from the condition.

An Integrated Approach to Understanding PCOS:

PCOS is frequently seen as a complex disorder having hormonal, metabolic, and lifestyle components. An integrated approach understands that effective management necessitates tackling all of these issues concurrently.

Integrated Medicine Approach Components:

An integrated medicine approach to PCOS includes a number of components that work together to address the problem holistically:

Medical Management: Traditional allopathic therapies, including hormone medication, lifestyle advice, and surgical procedures, are critical components of PCOS care. Endocrinologists and gynecologists that specialize in PCOS frequently administer these therapies.

Nutritional Advice: Integrative medicine practitioners frequently highlight the importance of diet in PCOS management. A licensed dietitian can assist people with PCOS in developing a well-balanced, low-glycemic diet that promotes blood sugar management and hormonal balance.

Mind-Body Techniques: Stress management is essential for PCOS. Yoga, meditation, and deep breathing are all mind-body techniques that can help decrease stress and enhance hormone balance.

There are specific breathing techniques again as per body type which I highly recommend. For example as a universal recommendation, gentle yogic stretch of all muscle groups and pelvic area are always welcome. Practices like anulom vilom, bhramari pranayam, and breath observation in moderation are all recommended for almost everyone. For those suffering from significant runny tummy or anxiety and fear kind of symptoms, left nostril breathing for 6-8 weeks only 10-20 min per day is recommended. Another very good breathwork practice is Wim Hoff Method for patients suffering from low energy and metabolic sluggishness, and symptoms of bloating and indigestion.

Acupuncture: In certain integrative medicine systems, acupuncture is used to stimulate particular acupoints associated with hormone management and menstrual cycle regularity.

There are specific acupoints around the calves and lower leg areas which your chiro or acupuncture can guide you to manipulate and stimulate on your own for better recovery.

Herbal and nutritional supplements: Some people with PCOS may benefit from herbs like chasteberry (Vitex agnus-castus) or nutritional supplements like inositol.

These should only be used with the supervision of a healthcare expert.

Inositol is my number one favorite, which works for almost all patients. For obese patients many polyherbal supplements like chandraprabha vati and single herbs are recommended, but it should never be self medicated, as these all are used as per body type. I strongly recommend here to always start even single herb supplements after consulting your integrative me specialist or an ayurvedic physician.

Exercise: Regular physical exercise can help you lose weight, increase insulin sensitivity, and regulate your menstrual cycle. Personalized fitness plans are frequently encouraged in integrative medicine.

Moderate exercise has been found to be most beneficial, too much and too little activity both can be detrimental. Exercising too much especially on a tired and sleep deprived body may drive up inflammation.

Functional Medicine: This method examines dietary inadequacies, hormone imbalances, and gut health to discover and treat the underlying causes of PCOS. Specialized testing and individualized treatment regimens may be used by a functional medicine practitioner.

Patient-Centered Care (PCC):

A patient-centered approach to PCOS is inherent in an integrated medicine approach. It acknowledges that each person's experience with PCOS is unique, and that treatment programs should be personalized to their specific requirements and goals. This method enables patients and healthcare practitioners to make decisions together.

Monitoring and Adjustment:

Regular monitoring of PCOS symptoms and associated health indicators is required to assess the efficacy of the combined treatment. Treatment programs can be modified as needed to achieve the greatest results for each person.

The Importance of Holistic Well-Being:
The integrated medicine approach acknowledges PCOS as a disorder that may have a significant impact on an individual's physical, emotional, and mental well-being. It promotes a comprehensive approach to health that includes:

- To treat the emotional burden of PCOS, emotional assistance and mental health services are available.
- A focus on self-care actions that increase happiness.

- Individuals are empowered to actively participate in their own health management.

Collaboration and communication:

The effectiveness of the integrated medicine strategy is dependent on collaboration among healthcare professionals. Effective communication and coordination among allopathic healthcare practitioners, dietitians, alternative therapists, and other experts engaged in the care of PCOS patients ensures that the patient receives a coherent and complete approach to therapy.

Finally, an integrated medicine approach to PCOS recognizes the condition's multidimensional character and blends standard medical treatments with complementary and alternative therapies. This approach is patient-centered, comprehensive, and adaptable, with the goal of improving not just the symptoms but also the general well-being of those with PCOS. It highlights the necessity of teamwork among healthcare practitioners as well as the patient's active participation in their own treatment. An integrated medicine approach to PCOS management provides a holistic method to managing this complicated disorder by addressing the physical, emotional, and mental elements of the problem.

Each lady with PCOS is different and the root causes may be completely different in each one of us. It should be evaluated very comprehensively and treatment fine tuned to individual needs.
TO KNOW YOUR BODY TYPE AND TO TAKE A COMPREHENSIVE QUESTIONNAIRE ABOUT YOUR AYURVEDIC BODY TYPE YOU MAY LIKE TO DOWNLOAD THE APP AIDOC AND ANALYZE YOUR OWN BODY TYPE, YOUR DOSA, THAT IS YOUR INNATE NATURE AND THE VIKRUTI THAT IS THE IMBALANCE OR AFFECTION CAUSING DISEASE.
YOU CAN SCAN THE QR CODE FOR THE APP.

CHAPTER 13- PSORIASIS

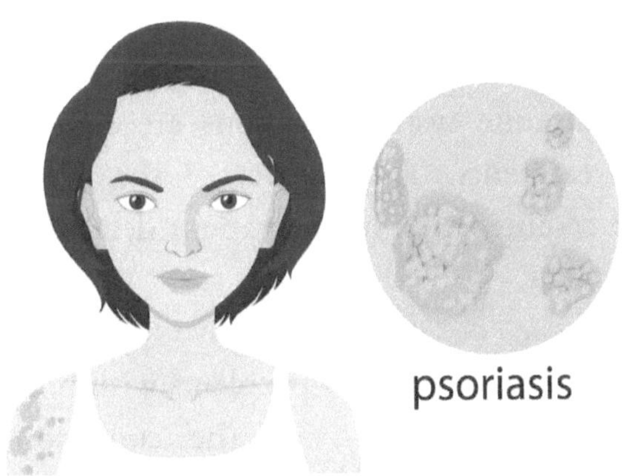

psoriasis

Psoriasis is a chronic skin disease that impacts millions of individuals globally. Skin cells proliferate quickly in this condition, resulting in the development of thick, red, scaly areas on the skin's surface. Although these so-called plaques can appear anywhere on the body, the elbows, knees, scalp, and lower back are the most often affected areas.

Although the precise etiology of psoriasis is unknown, a mix of environmental and genetic factors are thought to be responsible. Because the immune system misinterprets healthy skin cells as foreign invaders and overproduces skin cells in a defensive response, it plays a major role in the development of psoriasis.The typical plaques are caused by an irregular turnover of skin cells, which can also cause pain, irritation, and itching.

Although there is currently no known cure for psoriasis, there are a number of therapeutic options that can help manage its symptoms. Topical creams, laser therapy, oral medications, and biologic pharmaceuticals that specifically target immune system reactions are some examples of these treatments. The severity of the ailment and the unique requirements of the patient determine the course of treatment.

Psoriasis can be difficult to live with physically and psychologically because of problems with body image and self-esteem brought on by the condition's outward manifestation. Those with psoriasis may find that having a strong social network and medical support are essential.

Apart from its effects on the skin, psoriasis has been connected to many medical disorders such as metabolic syndrome, psoriatic arthritis, and cardiovascular disease. For this reason, it's critical that psoriasis patients collaborate closely with their medical professionals to identify and manage any possible comorbidities.

The detailed explanation of Psoriasis along with many other topics will be covered in the 2nd volume of this book. To know more about your body type log on to www.aiwell.in or download the app.

BIBLIOGRAPHY

1 . Koenig, H. G. et al. (2001). "Religious involvement and immune function in chronically ill, hospice, and healthy individuals."

2. Spijkerman, M. P. et al. (2016). "A meta-analysis of the efficacy of mindfulness-based stress reduction in behavior medicine settings."

3.Ingela C. Thuné-Boyle, Jan A. Stygall, Mohammed R. Keshtgar, Stanton P. Newman,
Do religious/spiritual coping strategies affect illness adjustment in patients with cancer? A systematic review of the literature,Social Science & Medicine,Volume 63, Issue 1,2006,Pages 151-164,ISSN 0277-9536,

4. Thune-Boyle, I. C. et al. (2006). "The role of spirituality in patients with chronic illness."

5. Büssing, A. et al. (2010). "Spirituality and adaptive coping style in German
patients with chronic diseases in a CAM health care setting."

6. Balboni, T. A. et al. (2007). "Religiousness, spiritual support, and patient perceptions of medical care at the end of life."

7. Sinclair, S. et al. (2006). "Cultural aspects of communication in cancer care."

8. Ehman, J. W. et al. (1999). "Do patients want physicians to inquire about their spiritual or religious beliefs if they become gravely ill?"

9. Stewart, M. E., and Downing, D. T. (1985), as cited. "Measurement of lipids in human skin, sebum, and comedones." 84(4), 335-338, Journal of Investigative Dermatology.

10. Leyden, J. J., et al. (1998). "The evolving role of Propionibacterium acnes in acne." Seminars in Cutaneous Medicine and Surgery, 17(3), 153-157.

11.Pagnoni, A., et al. (2001). "The role of follicular hyperkeratinization in acne." Journal of the American Academy of Dermatology, 45(3), S190-S194.

12. Thiboutot, D., et al. (2009). "Androgens and the skin." Endocrine Reviews, 29(5), 507-522.

13. Toyoda, M., & Morohashi, M. (2001). "Pathogenesis of acne." Medical Electron Microscopy, 34(1), 29-40.

14. Smith, R. N., et al. (2007). "A low-glycemic-load diet improves symptoms in acne vulgaris patients: a randomized controlled trial." The American Journal of Clinical Nutrition, 86(1), 107-115.
15. Bataille, V., et al. (2002). "Familial acne inversa: evidence of autosomal dominant inheritance." British Journal of Dermatology, 146(2), 240-242.

16. Chiu, A., Chon, S. Y., & Kimball, A. B. (2003). "The response of skin disease to stress: changes in the severity of acne vulgaris as affected by examination stress." Archives of Dermatology, 139(7), 897-900.

17. Shwereb, Christina, and Eve J Lowenstein. "Delayed type hypersensitivity to benzoyl peroxide." Journal of drugs in dermatology : JDD vol. 3,2 (2004): 197-9.

18. Hall JB, Cong Z, Imamura-Kawasawa Y, Kidd BA, Dudley JT, Thiboutot DM, Nelson AM. Isolation and Identification of the Follicular Microbiome: Implications for Acne Research. J Invest Dermatol. 2018 Sep;138(9):2033-2040

19. Li, Wen-Hwa et al. "Low-level red LED light inhibits hyperkeratinization and inflammation induced by unsaturated fatty acid in an in vitro model mimicking acne." Lasers in surgery and medicine vol. 50,2 (2018): 158-165. doi:10.1002/lsm.22747

20. Adebamowo CA, Spiegelman D, Danby FW, Frazier AL, Willett WC, Holmes MD. High school dietary dairy intake and teenage acne. J Am Acad Dermatol. 2005 Feb;52(2):207-14.

21.Thiboutot D. Acne: hormonal concepts and therapy. Clin Dermatol. 2004 Sep-Oct;22(5):419-28.

22. Cappel M, Mauger D, Thiboutot D. Correlation between serum levels of insulin-like growth factor 1, dehydroepiandrosterone sulfate, and dihydrotestosterone and acne lesion counts in adult women. Arch Dermatol. 2005 Mar;141(3):333-8

23. Holmes MD, Pollak MN, Willett WC, Hankinson SE. Dietary correlates of plasma insulin-like growth factor I and insulin-like growth factor binding protein 3 concentrations. Cancer Epidemiol Biomarkers Prev. 2002 Sep;11(9):852-61.
24. Spencer EH, Ferdowsian HR, Barnard ND. Diet and acne: a review of the evidence. Int J Dermatol. 2009 Apr;48(4):339-47.

25. Chiu, Annie et al. "The response of skin disease to stress: changes in the severity of acne vulgaris as affected by examination stress." Archives of dermatology vol. 139,7 (2003): 897-900. doi:10.1001/archderm.139.7.897

26. Yosipovitch G, Tang M, Dawn AG, Chen M, Goh CL, Huak Y, Seng LF. Study of psychological stress, sebum production and acne vulgaris in adolescents. Acta Derm Venereol. 2007;87(2):135-9.

27. Zhang M, Hu R, Huang Y, Zhou F, Li F, Liu Z, Geng Y, Dong H, Ma W, Song K, Song Y. Present and Future: Crosstalks Between Polycystic Ovary Syndrome and Gut Metabolites Relating to Gut Microbiota. Front Endocrinol (Lausanne). 2022 Jul 19;13:933110. doi: 10.3389/fendo.2022.933110. PMID: 35928893; PMCID: PMC9343597.

28. Kang W, Jang KH, Lim HM, Ahn JS, Park WJ. The menstrual cycle associated with insomnia in newly employed nurses performing shift work: a 12-month follow-up study. Int Arch Occup Environ Health. 2019;92(2):227–35

29. Kang W, Jang KH, Lim HM, Ahn JS, Park WJ. The menstrual cycle associated with insomnia in newly employed nurses performing shift work: a 12-month follow-up study. Int Arch Occup Environ Health. 2019 Feb;92(2):227-235. doi: 10.1007/s00420-018-1371-y. Epub 2018 Nov 1. PMID: 30386870.

30. Shoaibinobarian, Nargeskhatoon & Eslamian, Ghazaleh & Noormohammadi, Morvarid. (2022). Association between ultra-processed foods and polycystic ovary syndrome: a case-control study. 10.13140/RG.2.2.36013.97764.